Virtual Clinical Excursions—Medical-Surgical

for

Black and Hawks
Medical-Surgical Nursing:
Clinical Management for Positive Outcomes, 8th Edition

prepared by

Dorothy Mathers, RN, MSN
Associate Professor, Nursing
Pennsylvania College of Technology
Williamsport, Pennsylvania

software developed by

Wolfsong Informatics, LLC
Tucson, Arizona

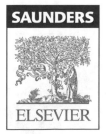

SAUNDERS

ELSEVIER

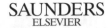

SAUNDERS
ELSEVIER

11830 Westline Industrial Dr.
St. Louis, Missouri 63146

VIRTUAL CLINICAL EXCURSIONS—MEDICAL-SURGICAL FOR
BLACK AND HAWKS: MEDICAL-SURGICAL NURSING:
CLINICAL MANAGEMENT FOR POSITIVE OUTCOMES,
EIGHTH EDITION

ISBN: 978-1-4160-5551-8

Notice

Knowledge and best practice in this field are constantly changing. As new research and experience broaden
our knowledge, changes in practice, treatment and drug therapy may become necessary or appropriate.
Readers are advised to check the most current information provided (i) on procedures featured or (ii) by the
manufacturer of each product to be administered, to verify the recommended dose or formula, the method
and duration of administration, and contraindications. It is the responsibility of the practitioner, relying on
their own experience and knowledge of the patient, to make diagnoses, to determine dosages and the best
treatment for each individual patient, and to take all appropriate safety precautions. To the fullest extent of
the law, neither the Publisher nor the Authors assumes any liability for any injury and/or damage to persons
or property arising out or related to any use of the material contained in this book.

ISBN: 978-1-4160-5551-8

Acquisitions Editor: *Jeff Downing*
Associate Developmental Editor: *Danny Witzofsky*
Project Manager: *Tracey Schriefer*

Working together to grow
libraries in developing countries

www.elsevier.com | www.bookaid.org | www.sabre.org

ELSEVIER   BOOK AID
            International   Sabre Foundation

Printed in the United States of America

Last digit is the print number: 9 8 7 6 5 4 3

*Workbook
prepared by*

Dorothy Mathers, RN, MSN
Associate Professor, Nursing
Pennsylvania College of Technology
Williamsport, Pennsylvania

Textbook

Joyce M. Black, PhD, RN, CPSN, CWCN, FAPWCA
Assistant Professor
College of Nursing
University of Nebraska Medical Center
Omaha, Nebraska

Jane Hokanson Hawks, DNSc, RN, BC
Associate Professor of Nursing
Midland Lutheran College
Fremont, Nebraska

Reviewers

Gina Long, RN, DNSc
Assistant Professor
Department of Nursing
College of Health Professions
Northern Arizona University
Flagstaff, Arizona

Diana Mixon, BSN, MSN
Associate Professor
Department of Nursing
Boise State University
Boise, Idaho

Contents

Unit 9—Circulatory Disorders

Unit 10—Oxygenation Disorders

Unit 11—Sensory Disorders

Unit 12—Cognitive and Perceptual Disorders

Unit 13—Protective Disorders

Table of Contents
Black and Hawks
Medical-Surgical Nursing:
Clinical Management for Positive Outcomes, 8th Edition

Getting Started

GETTING SET UP

■ MINIMUM SYSTEM REQUIREMENTS

WINDOWS®

Windows Vista™, XP, 2000 (Recommend Windows XP/2000)
Pentium® III processor (or equivalent) @ 600 MHz (Recommend 800 MHz or better)
256 MB of RAM (Recommend 1 GB or more for Windows Vista)
800 x 600 screen size (Recommend 1024 x 768)
Thousands of colors
12x CD-ROM drive
Soundblaster 16 soundcard compatibility
Stereo speakers or headphones

Note: Windows Vista and XP require administrator privileges for installation.

MACINTOSH®

MAC OS X (10.2 or higher)
Apple Power PC G3 @ 500 MHz or better
128 MB of RAM (Recommend 256 MB or more)
800 x 600 screen size (Recommend 1024 x 768)
Thousands of colors
12x CD-ROM drive
Stereo speakers or headphones

■ INSTALLATION INSTRUCTIONS

WINDOWS

1. Insert the *Virtual Clinical Excursions—Medical-Surgical* CD-ROM.
2. The setup screen should appear automatically if the current product is not already installed. Windows Vista users may be asked to authorize additional security prompts.
3. Follow the onscreen instructions during the setup process.

   If the setup screen does *not* appear automatically (and *Virtual Clinical Excursions—Medical-Surgical* has not been installed already):
   a. Click the **My Computer** icon on your desktop or on your Start menu.
   b. Double-click on your CD-ROM drive.
   c. If installation does not start at this point:
      (1) Click the **Start** icon on the taskbar and select the **Run** option.
      (2) Type d:\setup.exe (where "d:\" is your CD-ROM drive) and press **OK**.
      (3) Follow the onscreen instructions for installation.

MACINTOSH

1. Insert the *Virtual Clinical Excursions—Medical-Surgical* CD in the CD-ROM drive. The disk icon will appear on your desktop.

2. Double-click on the disk icon.

3. Double-click on the MEDICAL-SURGICAL_MAC run file.

Note: Virtual Clinical Excursions—Medical-Surgical for Macintosh does not have an installation setup and can only be run directly from the CD.

■ HOW TO USE VIRTUAL CLINICAL EXCURSIONS—MEDICAL-SURGICAL

WINDOWS

1. Double-click on the *Virtual Clinical Excursions—Medical-Surgical* icon located on your desktop.
2. Or navigate to the program via the Windows Start menu.

Note: If your computer uses Windows Vista, right-click on the desktop shortcut and choose **Properties**. In the Compatability Mode, check the box for "Run as Administrator." Below is a screen capture to show what this looks like.

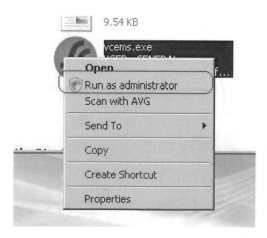

MACINTOSH

1. Insert the *Virtual Clinical Excursions—Medical-Surgical* CD in the CD-ROM drive. The disk icon will appear on your desktop.

2. Double-click on the disk icon.

3. Double-click on the MEDICAL-SURGICAL_MAC run file.

Note: Virtual Clinical Excursions—Medical-Surgical for Macintosh does not have an installation setup and can only be run directly from the CD.

■ SCREEN SETTINGS

For best results, your computer monitor resolution should be set at a minimum of 800 x 600. The number of colors displayed should be set to "thousands or higher" (High Color or 16 bit) or "millions of colors" (True Color or 24 bit).

Windows

1. From the **Start** menu, select **Control Panel** (on some systems, you will first go to **Settings**, then to **Control Panel**).
2. Double-click on the **Display** icon.
3. Click on the **Settings** tab.
4. Under **Screen resolution** use the slider bar to select **800 by 600 pixels**.
5. Access the **Colors** drop-down menu by clicking on the down arrow.
6. Select **High Color (16 bit)** or **True Color (24 bit)**.
7. Click on **OK**.
8. You may be asked to verify the setting changes. Click **Yes**.
9. You may be asked to restart your computer to accept the changes. Click **Yes**.

Macintosh

1. Select the **Monitors** control panel.
2. Select **800 x 600** (or similar) from the **Resolution** area.
3. Select **Thousands** or **Millions** from the **Color Depth** area.

■ WEB BROWSERS

Supported web browsers include Microsoft Internet Explorer (IE) version 6.0 or higher and Mozilla Firefox version 2.0 or higher. The supported browser for Macs running OS X is Mozilla Firefox.

If you use America Online® (AOL) for web access, you will need AOL version 4.0 or higher and one of the browsers listed above. Do not use earlier versions of AOL with earlier versions of IE, because you will have difficulty accessing many features.

For best results with AOL:
- Connect to the Internet using AOL version 4.0 or higher.
- Open a private chat within AOL (this allows the AOL client to remain open, without asking whether you wish to disconnect while minimized).
- Minimize AOL.
- Launch a recommended browser.

■ **TECHNICAL SUPPORT**

Technical support for this product is available between 7:30 a.m. and 7 p.m. (CST), Monday through Friday. Before calling, be sure that your computer meets the minimum system require-ments to run this software. Inside the United States and Canada, call 1-800-692-9010. Outside North America, call 314-872-8370. You may also fax your questions to 314-523-4932 or contact Technical Support through e-mail: technical.support@elsevier.com.

Trademarks: Windows, Macintosh, Pentium, and America Online are registered trademarks.

Copyright © 2009, 2006 by Saunders, an imprint of Elsevier Inc.

ACCESSING *Virtual Clinical Excursions—Medical-Surgical* FROM EVOLVE

The product you have purchased is part of the Evolve family of online courses and learning resources. Please read the following information thoroughly to get started.

To access your instructor's course on Evolve:

Your instructor will provide you with the username and password needed to access this specific course on the Evolve Learning System. Once you have received this information, please follow these instructions:

1. Go to the Evolve student page (http://evolve.elsevier.com/student).

2. Enter your username and password in the **Login to My Evolve** area and click the **Login** button.

3. You will be taken to your personalized **My Evolve** page, where the course will be listed in the **My Courses** module.

TECHNICAL REQUIREMENTS

To use an Evolve course, you will need access to a computer that is connected to the Internet and equipped with web browser software that supports frames. For optimal performance, it is recommended that you have speakers and use a high-speed Internet connection. However, slower dial-up modems (56 K minimum) are acceptable.

Whichever browser you use, the browser preferences must be set to enable cookies and JavaScript and the cache must be set to reload every time.

Enable Cookies

Browser	Steps
Internet Explorer (IE) 6.0 or higher	1. Select **Tools → Internet Options**. 2. Select **Privacy** tab. 3. Use the slider (slide down) to **Accept All Cookies**. 4. Click **OK**. -OR- 3. Click the **Advanced** button. 4. Click the check box next to **Override Automatic Cookie Handling**. 5. Click the **Accept** radio buttons under **First-party Cookies** and **Third-party Cookies**. 6. Click **OK**.
Mozilla Firefox 2.0 or higher	1. Select **Tools → Options**. 2. Select the **Privacy** icon. 3. Click to expand Cookies. 4. Select **Allow sites to set cookies**. 5. Click **OK**.

Set Cache to Always Reload a Page

Browser	Steps
Internet Explorer (IE) 6.0 or higher	1. Select **Tools → Internet Options**. 2. Select **General** tab. 3. Go to the **Temporary Internet Files** and click the **Settings** button. 4. Select the radio button for **Every visit to the page** and click **OK** when complete.
Mozilla Firefox 2.0 or higher	1. Select **Tools → Options**. 2. Select the **Privacy** icon. 3. Click to expand Cache. 4. Set the value to "**0**" in the **Use up to: __ MB of disk space for the cache** field. 5. Click **OK**.

Plug-Ins

 Adobe Acrobat Reader—With the free Acrobat Reader software, you can view and print Adobe PDF files. Many Evolve products offer student and instructor manuals, checklists, and more in this format!

Download at: http://www.adobe.com

 Apple QuickTime—Install this to hear word pronunciations, heart and lung sounds, and many other helpful audio clips within Evolve Online Courses!

Download at: http://www.apple.com

 Adobe Flash Player—This player will enhance your viewing of many Evolve web pages, as well as educational short-form to long-form animation within the Evolve Learning System!

Download at: http://www.adobe.com

 Adobe Shockwave Player—Shockwave is best for viewing the many interactive learning activities within Evolve Online Courses!

Download at: http://www.adobe.com

 Microsoft Word Viewer—With this viewer, Microsoft Word users can share documents with those who don't have Word, and users without Word can open and view Word documents. Many Evolve products have testbank, student and instructor manuals, and other documents available for downloading and viewing on your own computer!

Download at: http://www.microsoft.com

 Microsoft PowerPoint Viewer—With this viewer, you can access PowerPoint 97, 2000, and 2002 presentations even if you don't have PowerPoint. Many Evolve products have slides available for downloading and viewing on your own computer!

Download at: http://www.microsoft.com

SUPPORT INFORMATION

Live phone support is available to customers in the United States and Canada at **800-401-9962** from 7:30 a.m. to 7 p.m. (CST), Monday through Friday. Support is also available through email at evolve-support@elsevier.com.

Online 24/7 support can be accessed on the Evolve website (http://evolve.elsevier.com). Resources include:

- Guided tours
- Tutorials
- Frequently asked questions (FAQs)
- Online copies of course user guides
- And much more!

A QUICK TOUR

Welcome to *Virtual Clinical Excursions—Medical-Surgical*, a virtual hospital setting in which you can work with multiple complex patient simulations and also learn to access and evaluate the information resources that are essential for high-quality patient care. The virtual hospital, Pacific View Regional Hospital, has realistic architecture and access to patient rooms, a Nurses' Station, and a Medication Room.

■ BEFORE YOU START

Make sure you have your textbook nearby when you use the *Virtual Clinical Excursions—Medical-Surgical* CD. You will want to consult topic areas in your textbook frequently while working with the CD and using this workbook.

■ HOW TO SIGN IN

- Enter your name on the Student Nurse identification badge.
- Now choose one of the four periods of care in which to work. In Periods of Care 1 through 3, you can actively engage in patient assessment, entry of data in the electronic patient record (EPR), and medication administration. Period of Care 4 presents the day in review. Highlight and click the appropriate period of care. (For this quick tour, choose **Period of Care 1: 0730-0815**.)
- This takes you to the Patient List screen (see example on page 11). Only the patients on the Medical-Surgical Floor are available. Note that the virtual time is provided in the box at the lower left corner of the screen (0730, since we chose Period of Care 1).

Note: If you choose to work during Period of Care 4: 1900-2000, the Patient List screen is skipped since you are not able to visit patients or administer medications during the shift. Instead, you are taken directly to the Nurses' Station, where the records of all the patients on the floor are available for your review.

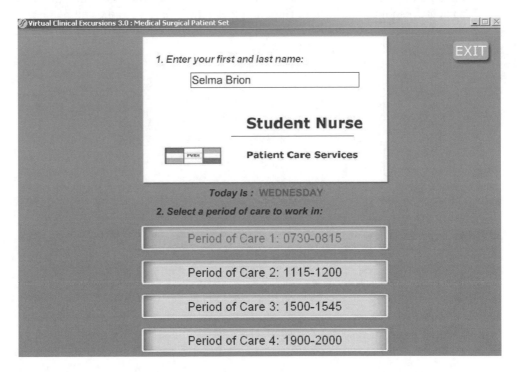

■ **PATIENT LIST**

MEDICAL-SURGICAL UNIT

Harry George (Room 401)

Osteomyelitis—A 54-year-old Caucasian male admitted from a homeless shelter with an infected leg. He has complications of type 2 diabetes mellitus, alcohol abuse, nicotine addiction, poor pain control, and complex psychosocial issues.

Jacquline Catanazaro (Room 402)

Asthma—A 45-year-old Caucasian female admitted with an acute asthma exacerbation and suspected pneumonia. She has complications of chronic schizophrenia, noncompliance with medication therapy, obesity, and herniated disc.

Piya Jordan (Room 403)

Bowel obstruction—A 68-year-old Asian female admitted with a colon mass and suspected adenocarcinoma. She undergoes a right hemicolectomy. This patient's complications include atrial fibrillation, hypokalemia, and symptoms of meperidine toxicity.

Clarence Hughes (Room 404)

Degenerative joint disease—A 73-year-old African-American male admitted for a left total knee replacement. His preparations for discharge are complicated by the development of a pulmonary embolus and the need for ongoing intravenous therapy.

Pablo Rodriguez (Room 405)

Metastatic lung carcinoma—A 71-year-old Hispanic male admitted with symptoms of dehydration and malnutrition. He has chronic pain secondary to multiple subcutaneous skin nodules and psychosocial concerns related to family issues with his approaching death.

Patricia Newman (Room 406)

Pneumonia—A 61-year-old Caucasian female admitted with worsening pulmonary function and an acute respiratory infection. Her chronic emphysema is complicated by heavy smoking, hypertension, and malnutrition. She needs access to community resources such as a smoking cessation program and meal assistance.

■ HOW TO SELECT A PATIENT

- You can choose one or more patients to work with from the Patient List by checking the box to the left of the patient name(s). For this quick tour, select Piya Jordan and Pablo Rodriguez. (In order to receive a scorecard for a patient, the patient must be selected before proceeding to the Nurses' Station.)
- Click on **Get Report** to the right of the medical records number (MRN) to view a summary of the patient's care during the 12-hour period before your arrival on the unit.
- After reviewing the report, click on **Go to Nurses' Station** in the right lower corner to begin your care. (*Note:* If you have been assigned to care for multiple patients, you can click on **Return to Patient List** to select and review the report for each additional patient before going to the Nurses' Station.)

Note: Even though the Patient List is initially skipped when you sign in to work for Period of Care 4, you can still access this screen if you wish to review the shift report for any of the patients. To do so, simply click on **Patient List** near the top left corner of the Nurses' Station (or click on the clipboard to the left of the Kardex). Then click on **Get Report** for the patient(s) whose care you are reviewing. This may be done during any period of care.

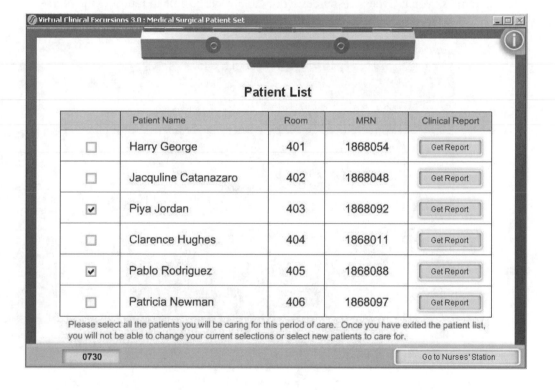

■ HOW TO FIND A PATIENT'S RECORDS

NURSES' STATION

Within the Nurses' Station, you will see:

1. A clipboard that contains the patient list for that floor.
2. A chart rack with patient charts labeled by room number, a notebook labeled Kardex, and a notebook labeled MAR (Medication Administration Record).
3. A desktop computer with access to the Electronic Patient Record (EPR).
4. A tool bar across the top of the screen that can also be used to access the Patient List, EPR, Chart, MAR, and Kardex. This tool bar is also accessible from each patient's room.
5. A Drug Guide containing information about the medications you are able to administer to your patients.
6. A tool bar across the bottom of the screen that can be used to access the Floor Map, patient rooms, Medication Room, and Drug Guide.

As you run your cursor over an item, it will be highlighted. To select, simply double-click on the item. As you use these resources, you will always be able to return to the Nurses' Station by clicking on the **Return to Nurses' Station** bar located in the right lower corner of your screen.

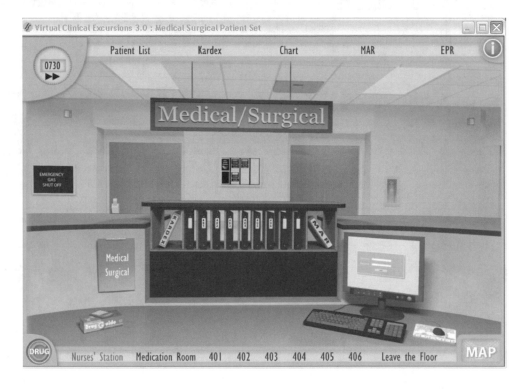

MEDICATION ADMINISTRATION RECORD (MAR)

The MAR icon located on the tool bar at the top of your screen accesses current 24-hour medications for each patient. Click on the icon and the MAR will open. (*Note:* You can also access the MAR by clicking on the MAR notebook on the far right side of the book rack in the center of the screen.) Within the MAR, tabs on the right side of the screen allow you to select patients by room number. Be careful to make sure you select the correct tab number for *your* patient rather than simply reading the first record that appears after the MAR opens. Each MAR sheet lists the following:

- Medications
- Route and dosage of each medication
- Times of administration of each medication

Note: The MAR changes each day. Expired MARs are stored in the patients' charts.

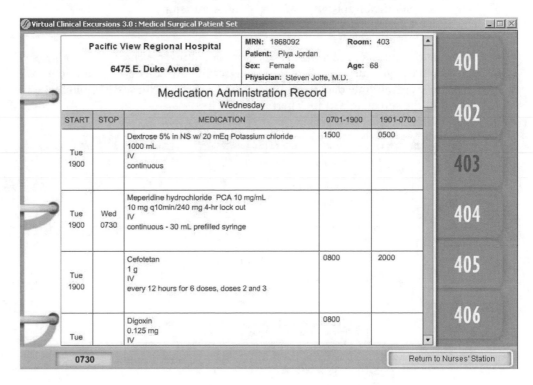

CHARTS

To access patient charts, either click on the **Chart** icon at the top of your screen or anywhere within the chart rack in the center of the Nurses' Station screen. When the close-up view appears, the individual charts are labeled by room number. To open a chart, click on the room number of the patient whose chart you wish to review. The patient's name and allergies will appear on the left side of the screen, along with a list of tabs on the right side of the screen, allowing you to view the following data:

- Allergies
- Physician's Orders
- Physician's Notes
- Nurse's Notes
- Laboratory Reports
- Diagnostic Reports
- Surgical Reports
- Consultations

- Patient Education
- History and Physical
- Nursing Admission
- Expired MARs
- Consents
- Mental Health
- Admissions
- Emergency Department

Information appears in real time. The entries are in reverse chronologic order, so use the down arrow at the right side of each chart page to scroll down to view previous entries. Flip from tab to tab to view multiple data fields or click on **Return to Nurses' Station** in the lower right corner of the screen to exit the chart.

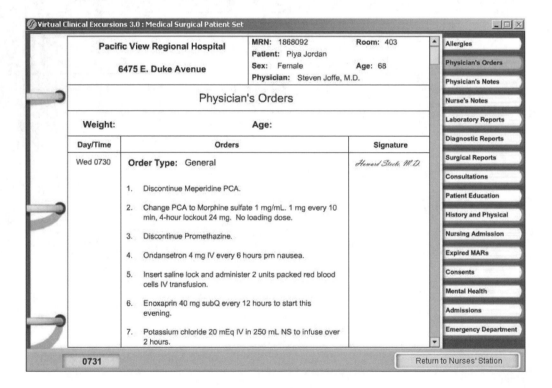

ELECTRONIC PATIENT RECORD (EPR)

The EPR can be accessed from the computer in the Nurses' Station or from the EPR icon located in the tool bar at the top of your screen. To access a patient's EPR:

- Click on either the computer screen or the **EPR** icon.
- Your username and password are automatically filled in.
- Click on **Login** to enter the EPR.
- *Note:* Like the MAR, the EPR is arranged numerically. Thus when you enter, you are initially shown the records of the patient in the lowest room number on the floor. To view the correct data for *your* patient, remember to select the correct room number, using the drop-down menu for the Patient field at the top left corner of the screen.

The EPR used in Pacific View Regional Hospital represents a composite of commercial versions being used in hospitals. You can access the EPR:

- to review existing data for a patient (by room number).
- to enter data you collect while working with a patient.

The EPR is updated daily, so no matter what day or part of a shift you are working, there will be a current EPR with the patient's data from the past days of the current hospital stay. This type of simulated EPR allows you to examine how data for different attributes have changed over time, as well as to examine data for all of a patient's attributes at a particular time. The EPR is fully functional (as it is in a real-life hospital). You can enter such data as blood pressure, breath sounds, and certain treatments. The EPR will not, however, allow you to enter data for a previous time period. Use the arrows at the bottom of the screen to move forward and backward in time.

Virtual Clinical Excursions 3.0 : Medical Surgical Patient Set				
Patient: 403 **Category:** Vital Signs				**0732**
Name: Piya Jordan	Wed 0630	Wed 0700	Wed 0715	Code Meanings
PAIN: LOCATION		OS		A — Abdomen
PAIN: RATING		5		Ar — Arm
PAIN: CHARACTERISTICS		C		B — Back
PAIN: VOCAL CUES		VC3		C — Chest
PAIN: FACIAL CUES		FC1		Ft — Foot
PAIN: BODILY CUES				H — Head
PAIN: SYSTEM CUES				Hd — Hand
PAIN: FUNCTIONAL EFFECTS				L — Left
PAIN: PREDISPOSING FACTORS				Lg — Leg
PAIN: RELIEVING FACTORS				Lw — Lower
PCA		P		N — Neck
TEMPERATURE (F)		99.6		NN — See Nurses notes
TEMPERATURE (C)				OS — Operative site
MODE OF MEASUREMENT		Ty		Or — See Physicians orders
SYSTOLIC PRESSURE		110		PN — See Progress notes
DIASTOLIC PRESSURE		70		R — Right
BP MODE OF MEASUREMENT		NIBP		Up — Upper
HEART RATE		104		
RESPIRATORY RATE		18		
SpO2 (%)		95		
BLOOD GLUCOSE				
WEIGHT				
HEIGHT				
◄		►		Exit EPR

At the top of the EPR screen, you can choose patients by their room numbers. In addition, you have access to 17 different categories of patient data. To change patients or data categories, click the down arrow to the right of the room number or category.

The categories of patient data in the EPR as as follows:

- Vital Signs
- Respiratory
- Cardiovascular
- Neurologic
- Gastrointestinal
- Excretory
- Musculoskeletal
- Integumentary
- Reproductive
- Psychosocial
- Wounds and Drains
- Activity
- Hygiene and Comfort
- Safety
- Nutrition
- IV
- Intake and Output

Remember, each hospital selects its own codes. The codes used in the EPR at Pacific View Regional Hospital may be different from ones you have seen in your clinical rotations. Take some time to acquaint yourself with the codes. Within the Vital Signs category, click on any item in the left column (e.g., Pain: Characteristics). In the far-right column, you will see a list of code meanings for the possible findings and/or descriptors for that assessment area.

You will use the codes to record the data you collect as you work with patients. Click on the box in the last time column to the right of any item and wait for the code meanings applicable to that entry to appear. Select the appropriate code to describe your assessment findings and type it in the box. (*Note:* If no cursor appears within the box, click on the box again until the blue shading disappears and the blinking cursor appears.) Once the data are typed in this box, they are entered into the patient's record for this period of care only.

To leave the EPR, click on **Exit EPR** in the bottom right corner of the screen.

■ VISITING A PATIENT

From the Nurses' Station, click on the room number of the patient you wish to visit (in the tool bar at the bottom of your screen). Once you are inside the room, you will see a still photo of your patient in the top left corner. To verify that this is the correct patient, click on the **Check Armband** icon to the right of the photo. The patient's identification data will appear. If you click on **Check Allergies** (the next icon to the right), a list of the patient's allergies (if any) will replace the photo.

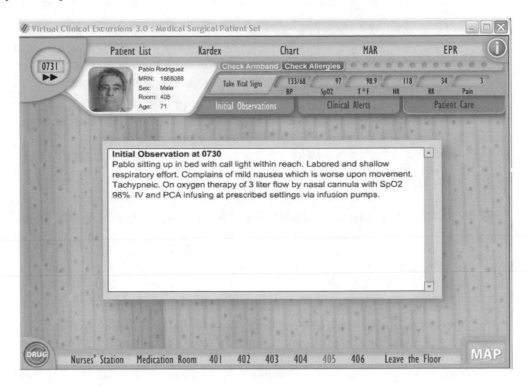

Also located in the patient's room are multiple icons you can use to assess the patient or the patient's medications. A virtual clock is provided in the upper left corner of the room to monitor your progress in real time. (*Note:* The fast-forward icon within the virtual clock will advance the time by 2-minute intervals when clicked.)

- The tool bar across the top of the screen allows you to check the **Patient List**, access the **EPR** to check or enter data, and view the patient's **Chart**, **MAR**, or **Kardex**.

- The **Take Vital Signs** icon allows you to measure the patient's up-to-the-minute blood pressure, oxygen saturation, temperature, heart rate, respiratory rate, and pain level.

- Each time you enter a patient's room, you are given an Initial Observation report to review (in the text box under the patient's photo). These notes are provided to give you a "look" at the patient as if you had just stepped into the room. You can also click on the **Initial Observations** icon to return to this box from other views within the patient's room. To the right of this icon is **Clinical Alerts**, a resource that allows you to make decisions about priority medication interventions based on emerging data collected in real time. Check this screen throughout your period of care to avoid missing critical information related to recently ordered or STAT medications.

- Clicking on **Patient Care** opens up three specific learning environments within the patient room: **Physical Assessment**, **Nurse-Client Interactions**, and **Medication Administration**.

- To perform a **Physical Assessment**, choose a body area (such as **Head & Neck**) from the column of yellow buttons. This activates a list of system subcategories for that body area (e.g., see **Sensory**, **Neurologic**, etc. in the green boxes). After you select the system you wish to evaluate, a brief description of the assessment findings will appear in a box to the right. A still photo provides a "snapshot" of how an assessment of this area might be done or what the finding might look like. For every body area, you can also click on **Equipment** on the right side of the screen.

- To the right of the Physical Assessment icon is **Nurse-Client Interactions**. Clicking on this icon will reveal the times and titles of any videos available for viewing. (*Note:* If the video you wish to see is not listed, this means you have not yet reached the correct virtual time to view that video. Check the virtual clock; you may return to access the video once its designated time has occurred—as long as you do so within the same period of care. Or you can click on the fast-forward icon within the virtual clock to advance the time by 2-minute intervals. You will then need to click again on **Patient Care** and **Nurse-Client Interactions** to refresh the screen.) To view a listed video, click on the white arrow to the right of the video title. Use the control buttons below the video to start, stop, pause, rewind, or fast-forward the action or to mute the sound.

- **Medication Administration** is the pathway that allows you to review and administer medications to a patient after you have prepared them in the Medication Room. This process is addressed further in the *How to Prepare Medications* section (pages 19-20) and in *Medications* (pages 26-30). For additional hands-on practice, see *Reducing Medication Errors* (pages 37-41).

■ HOW TO QUIT, CHANGE PATIENTS, OR CHANGE PERIODS OF CARE

How to Quit: From most screens, you may click the **Leave the Floor** icon on the bottom tool bar to the right of the patient room numbers. (*Note:* From some screens, you will first need to click an **Exit** button or **Return to Nurses' Station** before clicking **Leave the Floor**.) When the Floor Menu appears, click **Exit** to leave the program.

How to Change Patients or Periods of Care: To change patients, simply click on the new patient's room number. (You cannot receive a scorecard for a new patient, however, unless you have already selected that patient on the Patient List screen.) To change to a new period of care or to restart the virtual clock, click on **Leave the Floor** and then on **Restart the Program**.

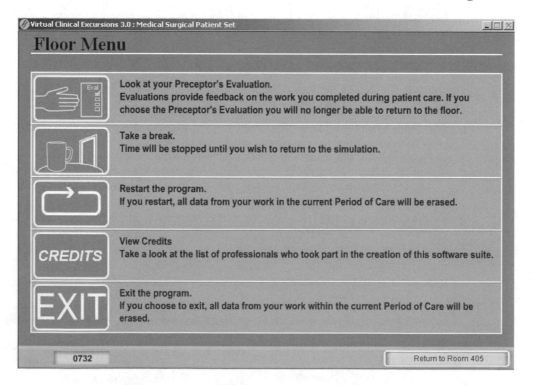

■ HOW TO PREPARE MEDICATIONS

From the Nurses' Station or the patient's room, you can access the Medication Room by clicking on the icon in the tool bar at the bottom of your screen to the left of the patient room numbers.

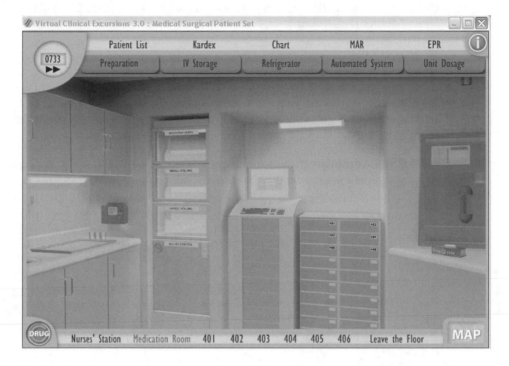

In the Medication Room you have access to the following (from left to right):

- A preparation area is located on the counter under the cabinets. To begin the medication preparation process, click on the tray on the counter or click on the **Preparation** icon at the top of the screen. The next screen leads you through a specific sequence (called the Preparation Wizard) to prepare medications one at a time for administration to a patient. However, no medication has been selected at this time. We will do this while working with a patient in *A Detailed Tour*. To exit this screen, click on **View Medication Room**.

- To the right of the cabinets (and above the refrigerator), IV storage bins are provided. Click on the bins themselves or on the **IV Storage** icon at the top of the screen. The bins are labeled **Microinfusion**, **Small Volume**, and **Large Volume**. Click on an individual bin to see a list of its contents. If you needed to prepare an IV medication at this time, you could click on the medication and its label would appear to the right under the patient's name. (*Note:* You can **Open** and **Close** any medication label by clicking the appropriate icon.) Next, you would click **Put Medication on Tray**. If you ever change your mind or decide that you have put the incorrect medication on the tray, you can reverse your actions by highlighting the medication on the tray and then clicking **Put Medication in Bin**. Click **Close Bin** in the right bottom corner to exit. **View Medication Room** brings you back to a full view of the entire room.

- A refrigerator is located under the IV storage bins to hold any medications that must be stored below room temperature. Click on the refrigerator door or on the **Refrigerator** icon at the top of the screen. Then click on the close-up view of the door to access the medications. When you are finished, click **Close Door** and then **View Medication Room**.

- To prepare controlled substances, click the **Automated System** icon at the top of the screen or click the computer monitor located to the right of the IV storage bins. A login screen will appear; your name and password are automatically filled in. Click **Login**. Select the patient for whom you wish to access medications; then select the correct medication drawer to open (they are stored alphabetically). Click **Open Drawer**, highlight the proper medication, and choose **Put Medication on Tray**. When you are finished, click **Close Drawer** and then **View Medication Room**.

- Next to the Automated System is a set of drawers identified by patient room number. To access these, click on the drawers or on the **Unit Dosage** icon at the top of the screen. This provides a close-up view of the drawers. To open a drawer, click on the room number of the patient you are working with. Next, click on the medication you would like to prepare for the patient, and a label will appear, listing the medication strength, units, and dosage per unit. To exit, click **Close Drawer**; then click **View Medication Room**.

At any time, you can learn about a medication you wish to prepare for a patient by clicking on the **Drug** icon in the bottom left corner of the medication room screen or by clicking the **Drug Guide** book on the counter to the right of the unit dosage drawers. The **Drug Guide** provides information about the medications commonly included in nursing drug handbooks. Nutritional supplements and maintenance intravenous fluid preparations are not included. Highlight a medication in the alphabetical list; relevant information about the drug will appear in the screen below. To exit, click **Return to Medication Room**.

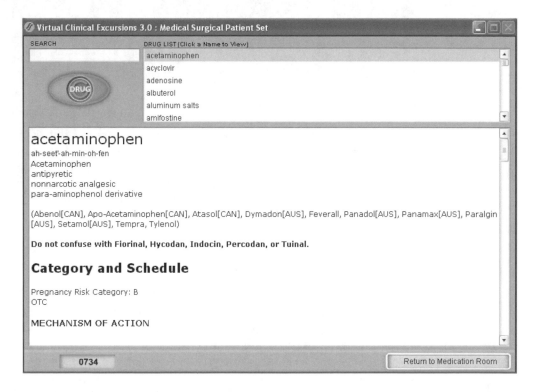

To access the MAR to review the medications ordered for a patient, click on the **MAR** icon located in the tool bar at the top of your screen and then click on the correct tab for your patient's room number. You may also click the **Review MAR** icon in the tool bar at the bottom of your screen from inside each medication storage area.

After you have chosen and prepared medications, go to the patient's room to administer them by clicking on the room number in the bottom tool bar. Inside the patient's room, click **Patient Care** and then **Medication Administration** and follow the proper administration sequence.

■ PRECEPTOR'S EVALUATIONS

When you have finished a session, click on **Leave the Floor** to go to the Floor Menu. At this point, you can click on the top icon (**Look at Your Preceptor's Evaluation**) to receive a scorecard that provides feedback on the work you completed during patient care.

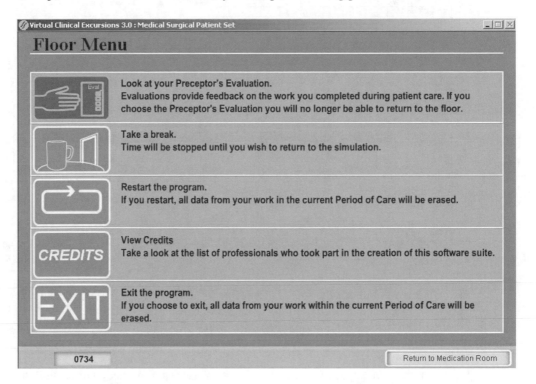

Evaluations are available for each patient you selected when you signed in for the current period of care. Click on the **Medication Scorecard** icon to see an example.

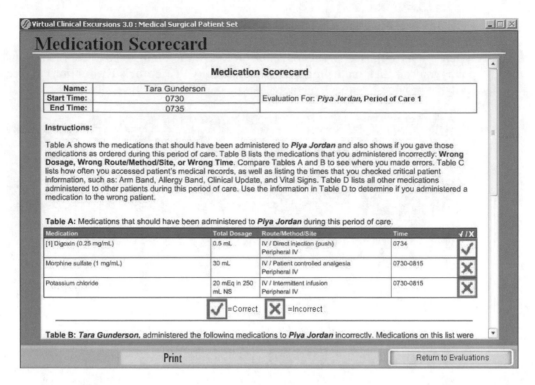

The scorecard compares the medications you administered to a patient during a period of care with what should have been administered. Table A lists the correct medications. Table B lists any medications that were administered incorrectly.

Remember, not every medication listed on the MAR should necessarily be given. For example, a patient might have an allergy to a drug that was ordered, or a medication might have been improperly transcribed to the MAR. Predetermined medication "errors" embedded within the program challenge you to exercise critical thinking skills and professional judgment when deciding to administer a medication, just as you would in a real hospital. Use all your available resources, such as the patient's chart and the MAR, to make your decision.

Table C lists the resources that were available to assist you in medication administration. It also documents whether and when you accessed these resources. For example, did you check the patient armband or perform a check of vital signs? If so, when?

You can click **Print** to get a copy of this report if needed. When you have finished reviewing the scorecard, click **Return to Evaluations** and then **Return to Menu**.

■ **FLOOR MAP**

To get a general sense of your location within the hospital, you can click on the **Map** icon found in the lower right corner of most of the screens in the *Virtual Clinical Excursions—Medical-Surgical* program. (*Note:* If you are following this quick tour step by step, you will need to **Restart the Program** from the Floor Menu, sign in again, and go to the Nurses' Station to access the map.) When you click the **Map** icon, a floor map appears, showing the layout of the floor you are currently on, as well as a directory of the patients and services on that floor. As you move your cursor over the directory list, the location of each room is highlighted on the map (and vice versa). The floor map can be accessed from the Nurses' Station, Medication Room, and each patient's room.

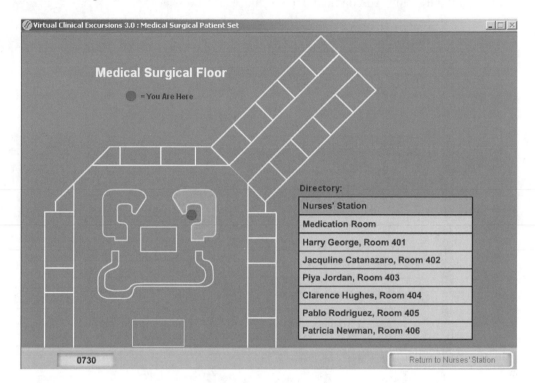

A DETAILED TOUR

If you wish to more thoroughly understand the capabilities of *Virtual Clinical Excursions—Medical-Surgical*, take a detailed tour by completing the following section. During this tour, we will work with a specific patient to introduce you to all the different components and learning opportunities available within the software.

■ WORKING WITH A PATIENT

Sign in for Period of Care 1 (0730-0815). From the Patient List, select Piya Jordan and Pablo Rodriguez; however, do not go to the Nurses' Station yet.

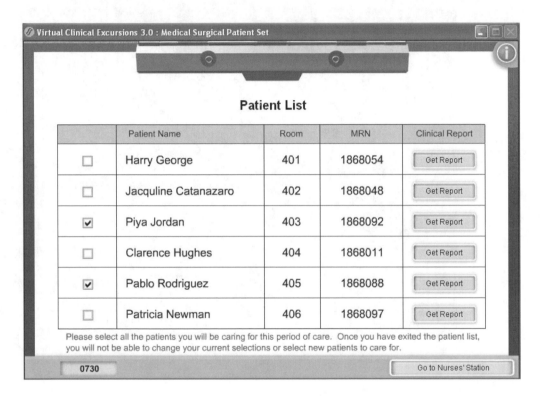

■ REPORT

In hospitals, when one shift ends and another begins, the outgoing nurse who attended a patient will give a verbal and sometimes a written summary of that patient's condition to the incoming nurse who will assume care for the patient. This summary is called a report and is an important source of data to provide an overview of a patient. Your first task is to get the clinical report on Piya Jordan. To do this, click **Get Report** in the far right column in this patient's row. From a brief review of this summary, identify the problems and areas of concern that you will need to address for this patient.

When you have finished noting any areas of concern, click **Go to Nurses' Station**.

■ CHARTS

You can access Piya Jordan's chart from the Nurses' Station or from the patient's room (403). From the Nurses' Station, click on the chart rack or on the **Chart** icon in the tool bar at the top of your screen. Next, click on the chart labeled **403** to open the medical record for Piya Jordan. Click on the **Emergency Department** tab to view a record of why this patient was admitted.

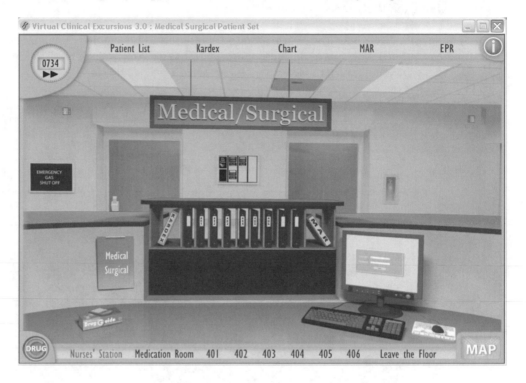

How many days has Piya Jordan been in the hospital?

What tests were done upon her arrival in the Emergency Department and why?

What was her reason for admission?

You should also click on **Surgical Reports** to learn what procedures were performed and when. Finally, review the **Nursing Admission** and **History and Physical** to learn about the health history of this patient. When you are done reviewing the chart, click **Return to Nurses' Station**.

■ MEDICATIONS

Open the Medication Administration Record (MAR) by clicking on the **MAR** icon in the tool bar at the top of your screen. *Remember:* The MAR automatically opens to the first occupied room number on the floor—which is not necessarily your patient's room number! Since you need to access Piya Jordan's MAR, click on tab **403** (her room number). Always make sure you are giving the *Right Drug to the Right Patient!*

Examine the list of medications ordered for Piya Jordan. In the table below, list the medications that need to be given during this period of care (0730-0815). For each medication, note the dosage, route, and time to be given.

Time	Medication	Dosage	Route

Click on **Return to Nurses' Station**. Next, click on **403** on the bottom tool bar and then verify that you are indeed in Piya Jordan's room. Select **Clinical Alerts** (the icon to the right of Initial Observations) to check for any emerging data that might affect your medication administration priorities. Next, go to the patient's chart (click on the **Chart** icon; then click on **403**). When the chart opens, select the **Physician's Orders** tab.

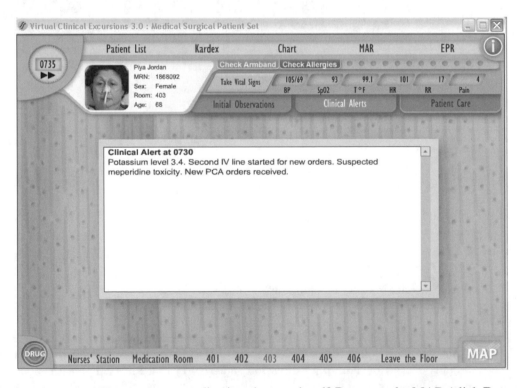

Review the orders. Have any new medications been ordered? Return to the MAR (click **Return to Room 403**; then click **MAR**). Verify that the new medications have been correctly transcribed to the MAR. Mistakes are sometimes made in the transcription process in the hospital setting, and it is sound practice to double-check any new order.

Are there any patient assessments you will need to perform before administering these medications? If so, return to Room 403 and click on **Patient Care** and then **Physical Assessment** to complete those assessments before proceeding.

Now click on the **Medication Room** icon in the tool bar at the bottom of your screen to locate and prepare the medications for Piya Jordan.

In the Medication Room, you must access the medications for Piya Jordan from the specific dispensing system in which each medication is stored. Locate each medication that needs to be given in this time period and click on **Put Medication on Tray** as appropriate. (*Hint:* Look in **Unit Dosage** drawer first.) When you are finished, click on **Close Drawer** and then on **View Medication Room**. Now click on the medication tray on the counter on the left side of the medication room screen to begin preparing the medications you have selected. (*Remember:* You can also click **Preparation** in the tool bar at the top of the screen.)

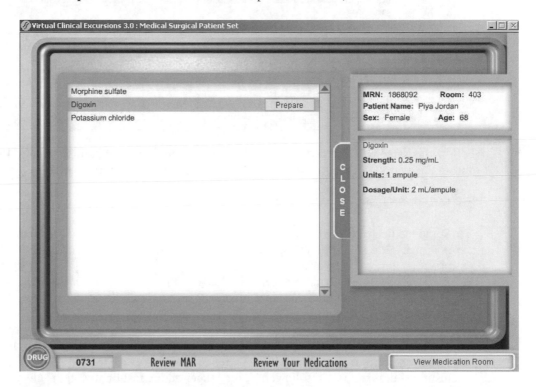

In the preparation area, you should see a list of the medications you put on the tray in the previous steps. Click on the first medication and then click **Prepare**. Follow the onscreen instructions of the Preparation Wizard, providing any data requested. As an example, let's follow the preparation process for digoxin, one of the medications due to be administered to Piya Jordan during this period of care. To begin, click to select **Digoxin**; then click **Prepare**. Now work through the Preparation Wizard sequence as detailed below:

> Amount of medication in the ampule: 2 mL.
> Enter the amount of medication you will draw up into a syringe: **0.5** mL.
> Click **Next**.
> Select the patient you wish to set aside the medication for: **Room 403, Piya Jordan**.
> Click **Finish**.
> Click **Return to Medication Room**.

Follow this same basic process for the other medications due to be administered to Piya Jordan during this period of care. (*Hint:* Look in **IV Storage** and **Automated System**.)

PREPARATION WIZARD EXCEPTIONS

- Some medications in *Virtual Clinical Excursions—Medical-Surgical* are preprepared by the pharmacy (e.g., IV antibiotics) and taken to the patient room as a whole. This is common practice in most hospitals.
- Blood products are not administered by students through the *Virtual Clinical Excursions— Medical-Surgical* simulations since blood administration follows specific protocols not covered in this program.
- The *Virtual Clinical Excursions—Medical-Surgical* simulations do not allow for mixing more than one type of medication, such as regular and Lente insulins, in the same syringe. In the clinical setting, when multiple types of insulin are ordered for a patient, the regular insulin is drawn up first, followed by the longer-acting insulin. Insulin is always administered in a special unit-marked syringe.

Now return to Room 403 (click on **403** on the bottom tool bar) to administer Piya Jordan's medications.

At any time during the medication administration process, you can perform a further review of systems, take vital signs, check information contained within the chart, or verify patient identity and allergies. Inside Piya Jordan's room, click **Take Vital Signs**. (*Note:* These findings change over time to reflect the temporal changes you would find in a patient similar to Piya Jordan.)

When you have gathered all the data you need, click on **Patient Care** and then select **Medication Administration**. Any medications you prepared in the previous steps should be listed on the left side of your screen. Let's continue the administration process with the digoxin ordered for Piya Jordan. Click to highlight **Digoxin** in the list of medications. Next, click on the down arrow to the right of **Select** and choose **Administer** from the drop-down menu. This will activate the Administration Wizard. Complete the Wizard sequence as follows:

- Route: **IV**
- Method: **Direct Injection**
- Site: **Peripheral IV**
- Click **Administer to Patient** arrow.
- Would you like to document this administration in the MAR? **Yes**
- Click **Finish** arrow.

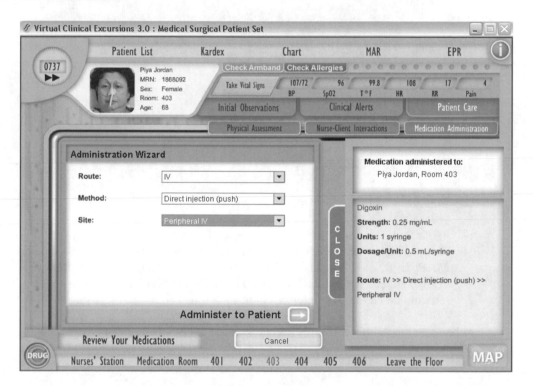

Your selections are recorded by a tracking system and evaluated on a Medication Scorecard stored under Preceptor's Evaluations. This scorecard can be viewed, printed, and given to your instructor. To access the Preceptor's Evaluations, click on **Leave the Floor**. When the Floor Menu appears, select **Look at Your Preceptor's Evaluation**. Then click on **Medication Scorecard** inside the box with Piya Jordan's name (see example on the following page).

■ MEDICATION SCORECARD

- First, review Table A. Was digoxin given correctly? Did you give the other medications as ordered?
- Table B shows you which (if any) medications you gave incorrectly.
- Table C addresses the resources used for Piya Jordan. Did you access the patient's chart, MAR, EPR, or Kardex as needed to make safe medication administration decisions?
- Did you check the patient's armband to verify her identity? Did you check whether your patient had any known allergies to medications? Were vital signs taken?

When you have finished reviewing the scorecard, click **Return to Evaluations** and then **Return to Menu**.

■ **VITAL SIGNS**

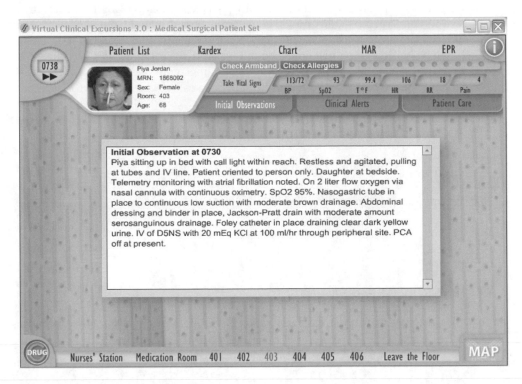

Vital signs, often considered the traditional "signs of life," include body temperature, heart rate, respiratory rate, blood pressure, oxygen saturation of the blood, and pain level.

Inside Piya Jordan's room, click **Take Vital Signs**. (*Note:* If you are following this detailed tour step by step, you will need to **Restart the Program** from the Floor Menu, sign in again, and navigate to Room 403.) Collect vital signs for this patient and record them below. Note the time at which you collected each of these data. (*Remember:* You can take vital signs at any time. The data change over time to reflect the temporal changes you would find in a patient similar to Piya Jordan.)

Vital Signs	Findings/Time
Blood pressure	
O$_2$ saturation	
Heart rate	
Respiratory rate	
Temperature	
Pain rating	

After you are done, click on the **EPR** icon located in the tool bar at the top of the screen. Your username and password are automatically provided. Click on **Login** to enter the EPR. To access Piya Jordan's records, click on the down arrow next to Patient and choose her room number, **403**. Select **Vital Signs** as the category. Next, in the empty time column on the far right, record the vital signs data you just collected in Piya Jordan's room. (*Note:* If you need help with this process, see page 16.) Now compare these findings with the data you collected earlier for this patient's vital signs. Use these earlier findings to establish a baseline for each of the vital signs.

    a.   Are any of the data you collected significantly different from the baseline for a particular vital sign?

        Circle One: Yes   No

    b.   If "Yes," which data are different?

■ PHYSICAL ASSESSMENT

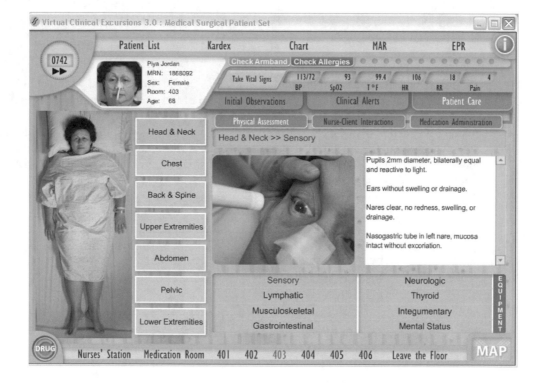

After you have finished examining the EPR for vital signs, click **Exit EPR** to return to Room 403. Click **Patient Care** and then **Physical Assessment**. Think about the information you received in the report at the beginning of this shift, as well as what you may have learned about this patient from the chart. Based on this, what area(s) of examination should you pay most attention to at this time? Is there any equipment you should be monitoring? Conduct a physical assessment of the body areas and systems that you consider priorities for Piya Jordan. For example, select **Head & Neck**; then click on and assess **Sensory** and **Lymphatic**. Complete any other assessment(s) you think are necessary at this time. In the following table, record the data you collected during this examination.

Area of Examination	Findings
Head & Neck Sensory	
Head & Neck Lymphatic	

After you have finished collecting these data, return to the EPR. Compare the data that were already in the record with those you just collected.

  a. Are any of the data you collected significantly different from the baselines for this patient?

     Circle One: Yes   No

  b. If "Yes," which data are different?

■ **NURSE-CLIENT INTERACTIONS**

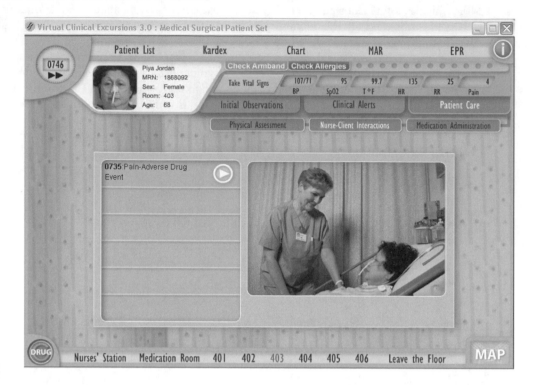

Click on **Patient Care** from inside Piya Jordan's room (403). Now click on **Nurse-Client Interactions** to access a short video titled **Pain—Adverse Drug Event**, which is available for viewing at or after 0735 (based on the virtual clock in the upper left corner of your screen; see *Note* below). To begin the video, click on the white arrow next to its title. You will observe a nurse communicating with Piya Jordan and her daughter. There are many variations of nursing practice, some exemplifying "best" practice and some not. Note whether the nurse in this interaction displays professional behavior and compassionate care. Are her words congruent with what is going on with the patient? Does this interaction "feel right" to you? If not, how would you handle this situation differently? Explain.

Note: If the video you wish to view is not listed, this means you have not yet reached the correct virtual time to view that video. Check the virtual clock; you may return to access the video once its designated time has occurred—as long as you do so within the same period of care. Or you can click on the fast-forward icon within the virtual clock to advance the time by 2-minute intervals. You will then need to click again on **Patient Care** and **Nurse-Client Interactions** to refresh the screen.

At least one Nurse-Client Interactions video is available during each period of care. Viewing these videos can help you learn more about what is occurring with a patient at a certain time and also prompt you to discern between nurse communications that are ideal and those that need improvement. Compassionate care and the ability to communicate clearly are essential components of delivering quality nursing care, and it is during your clinical time that you will begin to refine these skills.

■ COLLECTING AND EVALUATING DATA

Each of the activities you perform in the Patient Care environment generates a significant amount of assessment data. Remember that after you collect data, you can record your findings in the EPR. You can also review the EPR, patient's chart, videos, and MAR at any time. You will get plenty of practice collecting and then evaluating data in context of the patient's course.

Now, here's an important question for you:

> Did the previous sequence of exercises provide the most efficient way to assess Piya Jordan?

For example, you went to the patient's room to get vital signs, then back to the EPR to enter data and compare your findings with extant data. Next, you went back to the patient's room to do a physical examination, then again back to the EPR to enter and review data. If this back-and-forth process of data collection and recording seemed inefficient, remember the following:

- Plan all of your nursing activities to maximize efficiency, while at the same time optimizing the quality of patient care. (Think about what data you might need before performing certain tasks. For example, do you need to check a heart rate before administering a cardiac medication or check an IV site before starting an infusion?)

- You collect a tremendous amount of data when you work with a patient. Very few people can accurately remember all these data for more than a few minutes. Develop efficient assessment skills, and record data as soon as possible after collecting them.

- Assessment data are only the starting point for the nursing process.

Make a clear distinction between these first exercises and how you actually provide nursing care. These initial exercises were designed to involve you actively in the use of different software components. This workbook focuses on sensible practices for implementing the nursing process in ways that ensure the highest-quality care of patients.

Most important, remember that a human being changes through time, and that these changes include both the physical and psychosocial facets of a person as a living organism. Think about this for a moment. Some patients may change physically in a very short time (a patient with emerging myocardial infarction) or more slowly (a patient with a chronic illness). Patients' overall physical and psychosocial conditions may improve or deteriorate. They may have effective coping skills and familial support, or they may feel alone and full of despair. In fact, each individual is a complex mix of physical and psychosocial elements, and at least some of these elements usually change through time.

Thus it is crucial that you *DO NOT* think of the nursing process as a simple one-time, five-step procedure consisting of assessment, nursing diagnosis, planning, implementation, and evaluation. Rather, the nursing process should be utilized as a creative and systematic approach to delivering nursing care. Furthermore, because all living organisms are constantly changing, we must apply the nursing process over and over. Each time we follow the nursing process for an individual patient, we refine our understanding of that patient's physical and psychosocial conditions based on collection and analysis of many different types of data. *Virtual Clinical Excursions—Medical-Surgical* will help you develop both the creativity and the systematic approach needed to become a nurse who is equipped to deliver the highest-quality care to all patients.

REDUCING MEDICATION ERRORS

Earlier in this detailed tour, you learned the basic steps of medication preparation and administration. The following simulations will allow you to practice those skills further—with an increased emphasis on reducing medication errors by using the Medication Scorecard to evaluate your work.

Sign in to work at Pacific View Regional Hospital for Period of Care 1. (*Note:* If you are already working with another patient or during another period of care, click on **Leave the Floor** and then **Restart the Program**; then sign in.)

From the Patient List, select Clarence Hughes. Then click on **Go to Nurses' Station**. Complete the following steps to prepare and administer medications to Clarence Hughes.

- Click on **Medication Room**.
- Click on **MAR** and then on tab **404** to determine prn medications that have been ordered for Clarence Hughes. (*Note:* You may click on **Review MAR** at any time to verify the correct medication order. Always remember to check the patient name on the MAR to make sure you have the correct patient's record—you must click on the correct room number tab within the MAR.) Click on **Return to Medication Room** after reviewing the correct MAR.
- Click on **Unit Dosage** (or on the Unit Dosage cabinet); from the close-up view, click on drawer **404**.
- Select the medications you would like to administer. After each selection, click **Put Medication on Tray**. When you are finished selecting medications, click **Close Drawer** and then **View Medication Room**.
- Click on **Automated System** (or on the Automated System unit itself). Click **Login**.
- On the next screen, specify the correct patient and drawer location.
- Select the medication you would like to administer and click on **Put Medication on Tray**. Repeat this process if you wish to administer other medications from the Automated System.
- When you are finished, click **Close Drawer** and **View Medication Room**.
- From the Medication Room, click on **Preparation** (or on the preparation tray).
- From the list of medications on your tray, highlight the correct medication to administer and click **Prepare**.
- This activates the Preparation Wizard. Supply any requested information; then click **Next**.
- Now select the correct patient to receive this medication and click **Finish**.
- Repeat the previous three steps until all medications that you want to administer are prepared.
- You can click on **Review Your Medications** and then on **Return to Medication Room** when ready. Once you are back in the Medication Room, go directly to Clarence Hughes' room by clicking on **404** at bottom of screen.
- Inside the patient's room, administer the medication, utilizing the five rights of medication administration. After you have collected the appropriate assessment data and are ready for administration, click **Patient Care** and then **Medication Administration**. Verify that the correct patient and medication(s) appear in the left-hand window. Highlight the first medication you wish to administer; then click the down arrow next to Select. From the drop-down menu, select **Administer** and complete the Administration Wizard by providing any information requested. When the Wizard stops asking for information, click **Administer to Patient**. Specify **Yes** when asked whether this administration should be recorded in the MAR. Finally, click **Finish**.

■ **SELF-EVALUATION**

Now let's see how you did during your medication administration!

- Click on **Leave the Floor** at the bottom of your screen. From the Floor Menu, select **Look at Your Preceptor's Evaluation**. Then click **Medication Scorecard**.

The following exercises will help you identify medication errors, investigate possible reasons for these errors, and reduce or prevent medication errors in the future.

1. Start by examining Table A. These are the medications you should have given to Clarence Hughes during this period of care. If each of the medications in Table A has a √ by it, then you made no errors. Congratulations!

If any medication has an X by it, then you made one or more medication errors.

Compare Tables A and B to determine which of the following types of errors you made: Wrong Dose, Wrong Route/Method/Site, or Wrong Time. Follow these steps:
   a. Find medications in Table A that were given incorrectly.
   b. Now see if those same medications are in Table B, which shows what you actually administered to Clarence Hughes.
   c. Comparing Tables A and B, match the Strength, Dose, Route/Method/Site, and Time for each medication you administered incorrectly.
   d. Then, using the form below, list the medications given incorrectly and mark the errors you made for each medication.

Medication	Strength	Dosage	Route	Method	Site	Time
	❑	❑	❑	❑	❑	❑
	❑	❑	❑	❑	❑	❑
	❑	❑	❑	❑	❑	❑
	❑	❑	❑	❑	❑	❑

2. To help you reduce future medication errors, consider the following list of possible reasons for errors.

- Did not check drug against MAR for correct patient, correct date, correct time, correct drug, and correct dose.
- Did not check drug dose against MAR three times.
- Did not open the unit dose package in the patient's room.
- Did not correctly identify the patient using two identifiers.
- Did not administer the drug on time.
- Did not verify patient allergies.
- Did not check the patient's current condition or vital sign parameters.
- Did not consider why the patient would be receiving this drug.
- Did not question why the drug was in the patient's drawer.
- Did not check the physician's order and/or check with the pharmacist when there was a question about the drug or dose.
- Did not verify that no adverse effects had occurred from a previous dose.

Based on the list of possibilities you just reviewed, determine how you made each error and record the reason in the form below:

Medication	Reason for Error

3. Look again at Table B. Are there medications listed that are not in Table A? If so, you gave a medication to Clarence Hughes that he should not have received. Complete the following exercises to help you understand how such an error might have been made.

a. Perhaps you gave a medication that was on Clarence Hughes' MAR for this period of care, without recognizing that a change had occurred in the patient's condition, which should have caused you to reconsider. Review patient records as necessary and complete the following form:

Medication	Possible Reasons Not to Give This Medication

b. Another possibility is that you gave Clarence Hughes a medication that should have been given at a different time. Check his MAR and complete the form below to determine whether you made a Wrong Time error:

Medication	Given to Clarence Hughes at What Time	Should Have Been Given at What Time

c. Maybe you gave another patient's medication to Clarence Hughes. In this case, you made a Wrong Patient error. Check the MARs of other patients and use the form below to determine whether you made this type of error:

Medication	Given to Clarence Hughes	Should Have Been Given to

4. The Medication Scorecard provides some other interesting sources of information. For example, if there is a medication selected for Clarence Hughes but it was not given to him, there will be an X by that medication in Table A, but it will not appear in Table B. In that case, you might have given this medication to some other patient, which is another type of Wrong Patient error. To investigate further, look at Table D, which lists the medications you gave to other patients. See whether you can find any medications ordered for Clarence Hughes that were given to another patient by mistake. However, before you make any decisions, be sure to cross-check the MAR for other patients because the same medication may have been ordered for multiple patients. Use the following form to record your findings:

Medication	Should Have Been Given to Clarence Hughes	Given by Mistake to

5. Now take some time to review the medication exercises you just completed. Use the form below to create an overall analysis of what you have learned. Once again, record each of the medication errors you made, including the type of each error. Then, for each error you made, indicate specifically what you would do differently to prevent this type of error from occurring again.

Medication	Type of Error	Error Prevention Tactic

Submit this form to your instructor if required as a graded assignment, or simply use these exercises to improve your understanding of medication errors and how to reduce them.

Name: _____   Date: _____

The following icons are used throughout this workbook to help you quickly identify particular activities and assignments:

  Indicates a reading assignment—tells you which textbook chapter(s) you should read before starting each lesson

 Indicates a writing activity

 Marks the beginning of an interactive CD-ROM activity—signals you to open or return to your *Virtual Clinical Excursions—Medical-Surgical* CD-ROM

 Indicates additional CD-ROM instructions

 Indicates questions and activities that require you to consult your textbook

 Indicates the approximate time required to complete an exercise

Culturally Competent Care

/OTO **Reading Assignment:** Diversity in Health Care (available on Evolve Resources, Chapter 2)
Acute Health Care (Chapter 6, page 82)

Patients: Piya Jordan, Room 403
Clarence Hughes, Room 404
Pablo Rodriguez, Room 405

Goal: Demonstrate an understanding of the appropriate application of cultural concepts in nursing practice.

Objectives:

1. Define *culture* and associated terminology.
2. Explain methods of communicating with clients not fluent in English.
3. Identify appropriate methods of assessing the cultural needs of a client.
4. Describe nursing interventions relevant to meet the cultural needs of clients.
5. Correctly utilize the nursing process in providing culturally competent nursing care.

Overview:

In this lesson, you will assess the cultural needs of several clients and determine how nursing care might be adapted to meet each client's individual needs. Begin this activity by reviewing the general concepts presented in your textbook. Answer the following questions to solidify your understanding of culture.

Exercise 1

 Clinical Preparation: Writing Activity

20 minutes

1. Why is it important for a nurse to assess a client's culture?

2. Match each of the following terms with its correct definition or description.

Term	Definition or Description
_____ Culture	a. The belief that one's own beliefs and ways of doing things are the best
_____ Ethnicity	b. The learned and shared beliefs, values, and life-ways of a designated or particular group that are generally transmitted intergenerationally and influence one's thinking and action modes
_____ Ethnocentrism	c. A characteristic of groups in which a shared social and cultural heritage is passed on to each successive generation and in which there is a sense of identity

3. Identify the five cultural components pertinent to health care.

4. Describe six guidelines for the use of interpreters when communicating with clients not fluent in English.

5. How might you communicate with a non-English-speaking client if an interpreter was not available?

6. What is culturally competent care?

Exercise 2

 CD-ROM Activity

 45 minutes

- Sign in to work at Pacific View Regional Hospital for Period of Care 1. (*Note:* If you are already in the virtual hospital from a previous exercise, click on **Leave the Floor** and then **Restart the Program** to get to the sign-in window.)
- From the Patient List, select Piya Jordan (Room 403), Clarence Hughes (Room 404), and Pablo Rodriguez (Room 405).
- Click on **Go to Nurses' Station**.
- Click on **Chart** and then on **403**.
- Click on **History and Physical**.

1. Read Piya Jordan's History and Physical (H&P) and record her cultural needs and considerations in the table below and on the next page. Then repeat this process (using the last three steps above) for Clarence Hughes and Pablo Rodriguez to complete their sections of the table.

Client Name (Room Number)	Cultural Needs/Considerations
Piya Jordan (Room 403)	

Client Name (Room Number)	Cultural Needs/Considerations
Clarence Hughes (Room 404)	
Pablo Rodriguez (Room 405)	

 • Click on **Return to Nurses' Station**.
• Click on **403** to enter Piya Jordan's room.
• Read the **Initial Observations**.
• Click on **Patient Care** and then **Nurse-Client Interactions**.
• Select and view the video titled **0735: Pain—Adverse Drug Event**. (*Note:* Check the virtual clock to see whether enough time has elapsed. You can use the fast-forward feature to advance the time by 2-minute intervals if the video is not yet available. Then click again on **Patient Care** and **Nurse-Client Interactions** to refresh the screen.)

2. Based on this video, what potential cultural factors affecting health and health care should be identified and/or explored when planning care for Piya Jordan? (*Hint:* Use the general areas listed below to guide and organize your answers.)

Religion

Value Orientations

Health and Illness Beliefs

Communication

Family Roles and Lifestyle Patterns

- Click on **404** at the bottom of the screen to enter Clarence Hughes' room.
- Read the **Initial Observations**.
- Click on **Patient Care** and then **Nurse-Client Interactions**.
- Select and view the video titled **0730: Assessment/Perception of Care**. (*Note:* Check the virtual clock to see whether enough time has elapsed. You can use the fast-forward feature to advance the time by 2-minute intervals if the video is not yet available. Then click again on **Patient Care** and **Nurse-Client Interactions** to refresh the screen.)

3. Based on this video, what is Clarence Hughes' priority need at this time? What cultural factors affecting health and health care should the nurse explore when planning care specific for this need?

- Click on **405** at the bottom of the screen to enter Pablo Rodriguez's room.
- Read the **Initial Observations**.
- Click on **Patient Care** and then **Nurse-Client Interactions**.
- Select and view the video titled **0730: Symptom Management**. (*Note:* Check the virtual clock to see whether enough time has elapsed. You can use the fast-forward feature to advance the time by 2-minute intervals if the video is not yet available. Then click again on **Patient Care** and **Nurse-Client Interactions** to refresh the screen.)

4. Describe how Pablo Rodriguez's comments reveal his cultural beliefs.

LESSON *2*

Fluid Imbalance

✐ **Reading Assignment:** Clients with Fluid Imbalances (Chapter 11)

Patient: Piya Jordan, Room 403

Goal: Use the nursing process to competently care for clients with fluid imbalances.

Objectives:

1. Identify normal physiologic influences on fluid and electrolyte balance.
2. Compare and contrast the pathophysiology related to dehydration and overhydration.
3. Use laboratory data and clinical manifestations to assess fluid balance and imbalance.
4. Describe collaborative management strategies used to maintain and/or restore fluid balance.
5. Critically analyze fluid balance assessment findings in the assigned client.
6. Develop an appropriate plan of care for a client displaying a fluid imbalance.

Overview:

In this lesson you will assess, plan, and implement care for a client with an extracellular fluid imbalance. Piya Jordan is a 68-year-old female admitted with nausea and vomiting for several days following weeks of poor appetite and increasing weakness. You will begin this activity by reviewing the general concepts of fluid homeostasis as presented in your textbook. Answer the following questions to cement your understanding of the normal physiologic concepts related to fluid balance.

Exercise 1

Clinical Preparation: Writing Activity

30 minutes

1. Identify and describe the two major fluid compartments in the body.

2. Compare and contrast the causes and clinical manifestations of various types of fluid imbalances by completing the table below and on the next page.

Fluid Imbalance	Causes	Clinical Manifestations
Dehydration (extracellular fluid volume deficit [ECFVD])		
Cellular dehydration (intracellular fluid volume deficit)		
Fluid overload: hypervolemia (extracellular fluid volume excess [ECFVE])		

Fluid Imbalance	Causes	Clinical Manifestations
Water intoxication (intracellular fluid volume excess [ICFVE])		
Third space fluids (extracellular fluid volume shift)		

3. Describe the pathophysiology related to extracellular fluid volume deficit.

4. Identify and describe three types of extracellular fluid volume deficits.

Exercise 2

 CD-ROM Activity

 40 minutes

- Sign in to work at Pacific View Regional Hospital for Period of Care 1. (*Note:* If you are already in the virtual hospital from a previous exercise, click on **Leave the Floor** and then **Restart the Program** to get to the sign-in window.)
- From the Patient List, select Piya Jordan (Room 403).
- Click on **Go to Nurses' Station**.
- Click on **Chart** and then on **403** for Piya Jordan's chart.
- Click on **Emergency Department** and review this record.

1. Record findings below that support the diagnosis of dehydration for Piya Jordan.

 • Click on **Nursing Admission** and review.

2. Are there any additional findings noted on this document that support the diagnosis of dehydration? If so, list them below.

 3. Based on Piya Jordan's clinical manifestations, how would you classify the severity of her dehydration? Explain. (*Hint:* See Table 11-1 on page 130 of your textbook.)

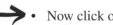 • Now click on and review the **Laboratory Reports**.

4. Below, record pertinent results noted on Piya Jordan's admission (Monday at 2200) and describe the significance of each result in relation to the diagnosis of dehydration.

 5. Calculate Piya Jordan's plasma osmolality, using the more accurate formula described on page 131 of your textbook.

 6. Based on the above findings, what type of fluid volume deficit do you think Piya Jordan is suffering from? (*Hint:* See page 129 of your textbook.) Explain.

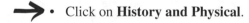 • Click on **History and Physical**.

7. What contributing factors led to Piya Jordan's dehydration?

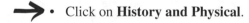 • Click on **Physician's Orders**.

8. Identify orders that are appropriate management strategies for the treatment of dehydration.

9. Below, develop an appropriate plan of care for Piya Jordan related to management of her fluid volume deficit.

Client Outcomes

Assessment Parameters

Collaborative Interventions

Electrolyte Imbalance, Part 1—Potassium

Reading Assignment: Clients with Electrolyte Imbalances (Chapter 12)

Patient: Piya Jordan, Room 403

Goal: Use the nursing process to competently care for clients with electrolyte imbalances.

Objectives:

1. Describe the effect of potassium imbalances on the action potential.
2. Identify specific etiologic factors related to hypokalemia for the assigned client.
3. Research potential drug interactions related to hypokalemia for the assigned client.
4. Assess the client for clinical manifestations related to hypo- and hyperkalemia.
5. Use the nursing process to correctly administer IV potassium chloride per physician's orders.

Overview:

In this lesson you will assess, plan, and implement care for a client with hypokalemia. Piya Jordan is a 68-year-old female admitted with nausea and vomiting for several days following weeks of poor appetite and increasing weakness. Begin this activity by reviewing the general functions of electrolytes within the body as presented in your textbook. Answer the following questions to cement your understanding of the normal physiologic concepts related to potassium balance.

Exercise 1

 Clinical Preparation: Writing Activity

 30 minutes

1. Cells use electrolytes for what two main purposes?

2. Describe the effect of potassium imbalance on the action potential.

3. Identify risk factors for hypokalemia.

4. Describe the clinical manifestations associated with hypokalemia. (*Hint:* Since these manifestations are numerous, organize your list by categories, such as symptoms that affect a particular body system, symptoms that affect a particular lab test, symptoms that occur as hypokalemia gets worse, etc.)

5. Identify causes and/or risk factors for hyperkalemia.

6. Describe the clinical manifestations associated with hyperkalemia.

Exercise 2

 CD-ROM Activity

  45 minutes

- Sign in to work at Pacific View Regional Hospital for Period of Care 1. (*Note:* If you are already in the virtual hospital from a previous exercise, click on **Leave the Floor** and then **Restart the Program** to get to the sign-in window.)
- From the Patient List, select Piya Jordan (Room 403).
- Click on **Go to Nurses' Station**.
- Click on **Chart** and then on **403**.
- Click on the **Laboratory Reports** tab.

1. What was Piya Jordan's initial potassium level on Monday at 2200?

 - Click on **Emergency Department** and review this record.

2. What would be the most likely cause for hypokalemia in this client?

3. What did the physician order to treat this electrolyte imbalance? Is this appropriate? (*Hint:* See page 153 of your textbook.)

4. Are the dilution and rate ordered by the physician safe to administer to Piya Jordan? Explain your answer. (*Hint:* If you need help, return to the Nurses' Station and click on the Drug Guide on the counter or click on the **Drug** icon in the bottom left corner of your screen.)

5. What should be assessed prior to administration of the KCl?

6. What precautions should be taken when administering the above IV solution of potassium?

• Click again on **Laboratory Reports**.

7. What was Piya Jordan's potassium level for Tuesday at 0630? Was the physician's order for potassium effective? Is there any cause for concern?

 • Click on **Return to Nurses' Station**.
• Click on **403** to go to the client's room.
• Click on **Patient Care** and then **Physical Assessment**.

8. Complete a physical assessment on Piya Jordan, specifically looking for clinical manifestations of hypokalemia. Document your findings in the chart below and the on the next page and underline those that correlate with hypokalemia.

Areas Assessed	Findings on Physical Exam
Cardiovascular	
Respiratory	
Neuromuscular	
Gastrointestinal	

Areas Assessed	Findings on Physical Exam
Renal	

9. What is the potassium level that was drawn on Wednesday at 0630?

10. Explain the etiology for this recurrence of hypokalemia.

- Click on **Chart** and then **403**.
- Click on **Physician's Orders**.

11. What did the physician order for Piya Jordan in response to today's potassium level?

Before administering KCl, you will need to assess Piya Jordan's renal status for adequate urine output.

- Click on **Return to Nurses'** Station.
- Click on **EPR** and then on **Login**.
- Choose **403** from the Patient drop-down menu. Select **Vital Signs** from the Category menu.

12. What is Piya Jordan's most recent weight?

13. What was Piya Jordan's urinary output from 11 p.m. Tuesday to 7 a.m. Wednesday? Is this adequate to infuse KCl?

Prepare to administer this ordered dose of potassium chloride to Piya Jordan by completing the following steps.

Medication Preparation

- Click on **Return to Room 403**.
- Click **Medication Room** on the bottom of your screen.
- Click on **IV Storage** near the top of your screen (*Note:* You can also click on any of the three bins just above the refrigerator.) Either of these methods will bring up a close-up view of the IV storage bins.
- Click on the bin labeled **Small Volume** and review the list of available medications. (*Note:* You may click on **Review MAR** at any time to verify correct medication order. Remember to look at the patient name on the MAR to make sure you have the correct patient's record—you must click on the correct room number within the MAR. Click on **Return to Medication Room** after reviewing the correct MAR.)
- From the list of medications in the bin, select **potassium chloride**. Then click **Put Medication on Tray** and **Close Bin**.
- Click **View Medication Room**.
- Click on **Preparation** at the top of the screen or on the preparation tray on the counter. Select the correct medication to administer; then click **Prepare**.
- Wait for instructions or questions from the Preparation Wizard. Then click **Next**.
- Choose the correct patient to administer this medication to. Click **Finish**.
- You can click **Review Your Medications** and then **Return to Medication Room** when ready. From the Medication Room, go directly to Piya Jordan's room by clicking on **403** at the bottom of the screen.

Prior to administering intravenous medications, the client's IV site must first be assessed.

- Click on **Patient Care**.
- Click on **Upper Extremities**.
- Select **Integumentary** from the system subcategories.

14. Document Piya Jordan's IV site assessment findings below. Is it appropriate to administer the IV potassium at this time?

Medication Administration

- After you have collected the appropriate assessment data and are ready for administration, click on **Medication Administration**.
- To the right of the medication name, next to Select, click the down arrow and choose **Administer** from the drop-down menu.
- Complete the Administration Wizard and click **Administer to Patient** when done.
- Check **Yes** when asked whether this drug administration should be documented on the MAR. Then click **Finish**.

→ • Now click on **MAR** at the top of your screen.

15. Look at Piya Jordan's MAR. What are her scheduled AM medications? What medication(s) would you question giving? Why?

16. For what clinical manifestations of digitalis toxicity should the nurse monitor Piya Jordan?

Now let's see how you did with your medication preparation and administration!

→ • Click on **Leave the Floor** at the bottom of your screen.
   • From the Floor Menu, select **Look at Your Preceptor's Evaluation**.
   • Then click on **Medication Scorecard** for Piya Jordan.

17. Disregard the report for the routine scheduled medications, but note whether or not you correctly administered the potassium chloride. If not, why do you think you were incorrect in administering this drug? According to Table C in this scorecard, what are the appropriate resources that should be used and important assessments that should be completed prior to administering this medication? Did you use these resources and perform these assessments correctly?

Electrolyte Imbalance, Part 2—Calcium, Phosphate, and Sodium

/O𝒷𝒷 **Reading Assignment:** Clients with Fluid Imbalances (Chapter 11)
Clients with Electrolyte Imbalances (Chapter 12)

Patient: Pablo Rodriguez, Room 405

Goal: Use the nursing process to competently care for clients with electrolyte imbalances.

Objectives:

1. Describe the pathophysiologic basis of electrolyte imbalances noted on a specific client.
2. Identify specific etiologic factor(s) related to hypercalcemia, hyponatremia, and hypophosphatemia in the assigned client.
3. Assess the assigned client for clinical manifestations related to sodium, calcium, and phosphorus imbalances.
4. Describe nursing interventions appropriate when caring for a client with hypercalcemia, hyponatremia, and hypophosphatemia.
5. Evaluate the effectiveness of medications prescribed to treat electrolyte imbalances.

Overview:

In this lesson you will assess, plan, and implement care for a client with several electrolyte imbalances. Pablo Rodriguez is a 71-year-old male who is admitted after experiencing nausea and vomiting for several days. He has a 1-year history of lung carcinoma. Begin this activity by reviewing the general functions of specific electrolytes within the body as presented in your textbook. Answer the following questions to cement your understanding of the physiologic concepts related to phosphate, sodium, and calcium imbalance.

Exercise 1

Clinical Preparation: Writing Activity

15 minutes

1. Prior to caring for a client with multiple electrolyte imbalances, it is imperative that you first review and reinforce general concepts related to specific electrolytes. Using the textbook, complete the table below by providing information related to specific calcium, phosphorus, and sodium imbalances. Refer to this table as you proceed through the CD-ROM activity to relate textbook knowledge to actual client care.

Electrolyte Imbalance	Diagnostic Lab Value	Etiology and Risk Factors	Pathophysiology
Hypercalcemia	Higher than 5.5 mEq/L or 11.0 mg/dL		
Hypophosphatemia	Less than 1.2 mEq/L or 2.8 mg/dL		
Hyponatremia	Less than 135 mEq/L		

Exercise 2

 CD-ROM Activity

 45 minutes

- Sign in to work at Pacific View Regional Hospital for Period of Care 1. (*Note:* If you are already in the virtual hospital from a previous exercise, click on **Leave the Floor** and then **Restart the Program** to get to the sign-in window.)
- From the Patient List, select Pablo Rodriguez (Room 405).
- Click on **Go to Nurses' Station**.
- Click on **Chart** and then **405**.
- Click on **Laboratory Reports**.

1. Record Pablo Rodriguez's serum chemistry results in the table below. Identify abnormal values by marking as H (for high) or L (for low). (*Hint:* Lab value results for calcium, phosphorus, and magnesium are measured in mg/dL.)

Lab Test	Results, Tuesday 2000	Results, Wednesday 0730
Sodium		
Potassium		
Calcium		
Phosphorus		
Magnesium		
Glucose		
BUN		
Hematocrit		

→ - Click on **Emergency Department**.

2. What would be the most likely cause for the hyponatremia noted in Pablo Rodriguez on admission?

3. What did the physician order to treat this electrolyte imbalance?

4. What was Pablo Rodriguez's sodium level for Wednesday at 0730? Was the physician's ordered treatment effective? Can you anticipate or suggest any change in orders?

5. Hyponatremia can be associated with both hypovolemia (actual sodium loss) and hyper-volumia (dilutional). Based on Pablo Rodriguez's presentation to the emergency depart-ment, what type of hyponatremia do you think he is experiencing? Explain.

- Click on **Return to Nurses' Station**.
- Click on **EPR** and then on **Login**.
- Select **405** as the Patient and **Intake and Output** as the Category.

6. Record the I&O shift totals for Pablo Rodriguez below.

Shift Totals	Tuesday 0705	Tuesday 1505	Tuesday 2305	Wednesday 0705
Intake				
Output				

7. Based on the above I&O totals obtained after the client received IV replacement therapy, what factor(s) may be contributing to the persistant hyponatremia? Explain your answer.

8. What other lab test might be useful to more accurately determine Pablo Rodriguez's hydration status? (*Hint:* See page 138 of your textbook.)

 9. Calculate the client's plasma osmolality based on his lab results for Wednesday at 0730. (*Hint:* Use the more exact formula noted on page 131 of your textbook.)

10. What do the results noted in questions 1 and 9 tell you about Pablo Rodriguez's fluid volume status?

 • Click on **Exit EPR**.
   • Click on **405** to go to the client's room.
   • Click on **Patient Care** and then **Physical Assessment**.

 11. Complete a physical assessment on Pablo Rodriguez, specifically looking for clinical manifestations of hyponatremia. (*Hint:* Refer to page 144 in your textbook.) Document your findings in the table below and on the next page and underline those that correlate with hyponatremia.

Areas Assessed	Findings on Physical Examination
Cardiovascular	
Respiratory	

Areas Assessed	Findings on Physical Examination
Neuromuscular	
Gastrointestinal	

→ • Click on **Chart** and then **405**.
   • Click on **Nursing Admission**.

12. Review the findings that you underlined in question 11. What other factors noted on the Nursing Admission form could be causing or contributing to these manifestations?

13. Based on your answer to the last two questions, what conclusion can you make regarding these clinical manifestations and Pablo Rodriguez's sodium levels?

 14. What other clinical manifestations of hyponatremia might you expect to find in other clients with this electrolyte imbalance? (*Hint:* See page 144 in your textbook.)

15. If Pablo Rodriguez had a sodium level of 115 mEq/L (severe hyponatremia), how would the treatment vary?

Exercise 3

 CD-ROM Activity

 60 minutes

- Sign in to work at Pacific View Regional Hospital for Period of Care 3. (*Note:* If you are already in the virtual hospital from a previous exercise, click on **Leave the Floor** and then **Restart the Program** to get to the sign-in window.)
- From the Patient List, select Pablo Rodriguez (Room 405).
- Click on **Go to Nurses' Station**.
- Click on **Chart** and then on **405** for Pablo Rodriguez's chart.
- Click on the **History and Physical**.

1. What electrolyte imbalances did Pablo Rodriguez present with on admission?

→ • Click on **Laboratory Reports**.

2. What was Pablo Rodriguez's calcium level on admission to the ED on Tuesday evening?

3. How does this level correlate with the physician's diagnosis? Speculate as to the reason for the discrepancy.

4. What was Pablo Rodriguez's phosphorus level during the same time period?

5. How does this relate to his calcium level?

➡ • Click on **History and Physical**.

6. What would be the most likely cause for hypercalcemia in this client?

➡ • Click on **Physician's Orders**.

7. What medication did the ED physician order to treat the hypercalcemia?

➡ • Click on **Return to Nurses' Station**.
   • Then click on either the Drug Guide on the counter or the **Drug** icon in the bottom left corner of your screen.

8. Describe the mechanism of action and therapeutic effect of the medication you identified in question 7.

9. What nursing assessments are appropriate related to the administration of this medication?

→ • Click on **Return to Nurses' Station**.
  • Click on **Chart** and then on **405**.
  • Click on **Laboratory Reports**.

10. What were Pablo Rodriguez's calcium and phosphorus levels this morning (Wednesday at 0730)?

11. Was the prescribed medication effective? Is the client out of danger?

→ • Click on **Return to Nurses' Station**.
  • Click on **Kardex** and then on tab **405**.

12. What intravenous fluids is Pablo Rodriguez receiving?

13. What is the purpose of IV hydration in relation to serum calcium levels?

14. Is this the solution you would normally expect to administer to a client with hypercalcemia? If not, what solution would you expect and why?

→ • Click on **Return to Nurses' Station**.
  • Click on **MAR** and then on tab **405**.

15. What medication is scheduled to be administered at 1500?

16. What electrolyte imbalance will this medication correct? Explain your answer. (*Hint:* Consult the Drug Guide in the Nurses' Station.)

17. What nursing assessments must be completed prior to administering this drug?

18. Do you have any concerns regarding administering this drug at this time? (*Hint:* Review the client's GI history on admission in the chart.)

→ • Click on **Return to Nurses' Station** and then on **405**.
   • Click on **Patient Care** and then **Physical Assessment**.

19. Complete a physical assessment on Pablo Rodriguez (including vital signs). Document your findings below and on the next page.

Areas Assessed	Findings on Physical Examination
Cardiovascular	
Respiratory	

Areas Assessed	Findings on Physical Examination
Neuromuscular	
Gastrointestinal	

20. Is Pablo Rodriguez demonstrating any clinical manifestations of hypercalcemia? If yes, describe the pathophysiologic basis for the symptoms. If not, explain why not.

 21. If Pablo Rodriguez had a calcium level of 13.5, what other clinical manifestations might you expect to find? (*Hint:* See page 162 in the textbook.)

22. When evaluating Pablo Rodriguez's renal output, what potential complication(s) of hypercalcemia would you be alert for?

23. Which foods would you teach Pablo Rodriguez to avoid based on his electrolyte imbalance?

24. After successful treatment of Pablo Rodriguez, the nurse must be alert for overcorrecting of the electrolyte imbalance. For what clinical manifestations should the nurse monitor this client related to hypocalcemia and hyperphosphatemia?

LESSON 5

Acid-Base Imbalance

📖 **Reading Assignment:** Acid-Base Balance (Chapter 13)

Patient: Jacquline Catanazaro, Room 402

Goal: Use the nursing process to competently care for clients with acid-base imbalances.

Objectives:

1. Describe the pathophysiologic basis of acid-base imbalance noted in the assigned client.
2. Identify specific etiologic factor(s) related to respiratory acidosis in the assigned client.
3. Assess the assigned client for clinical manifestations related to respiratory acidosis.
4. Describe nursing interventions appropriate when caring for a client with respiratory |acidosis.
5. Evaluate the effectiveness of medication prescribed to treat acid-base imbalances.

Overview:

In this lesson you will assess, plan, and implement care for a client with an acid-base imbalance. Jacquline Catanazaro is a 45-year-old female admitted with exacerabation of asthma and schizophrenia. Begin this lesson by reviewing the general concepts of acid-base balance as presented in your textbook.

Exercise 1

 Clinical Preparation: Writing Activity

 20 minutes

1. Define or provide the correct lab value/range for each of the following terms.

   a. pH

b. Normal serum pH

c. Neutral pH

d. Acidic solution

e. Alkaline solution

2. Identify and describe the three physiologic systems that work to maintain acid-base home-ostasis by completing the following table.

System	Mechanisms of Action	Acid-Base Compensation

Exercise 2

  CD-ROM Activity

45 minutes

- Sign in to work at Pacific View Regional Hospital for Period of Care 1. (*Note:* If you are already in the virtual hospital from a previous exercise, click on **Leave the Floor** and then **Restart the Program** to get to the sign-in window.)
- From the Patient List, select Jacquline Catanazaro (Room 402).
- Click on **Go to Nurses' Station**.
- Click on **Chart** and then on **402**.
- Click on **History and Physical**.

1. Is there anything in Jacquline Catanazaro's history that would put her at risk for an acid-base imbalance? Explain.

- Click on **Return to Nurses' Station** and then on **402**.
- Click on **Patient Care** and then **Nurse-Client Interactions**.
- Select and view the video titled **0730: Intervention—Airway**. (*Note:* Check the virtual clock to see whether enough time has elapsed. You can use the fast-forward feature to advance the time by 2-minute intervals if the video is not yet available. Then click again on **Patient Care** and **Nurse-Client Interactions** to refresh the screen.)

2. Based on Jacquline Catanazaro's history, what would you expect to be causing her respiratory distress?

3. Why is the nurse waiting until after the ABGs are drawn to give the client a nebulizer treatment?

- Click on **Chart** and then on **402**.
- Click on **Laboratory Reports**.

4. What are the results of Jacquline Catanazaro's two most recent ABGs? Document these results in the table below.

Results	Monday 1030	Wednesday 0730
pH		
PaO_2		
$PaCO_2$		
O_2 sat		
Bicarb		

5. How would you interpret the above results? Is the acid-base imbalance compensated or uncompensated (fully or partially)? Explain your answer.

6. Based on the acute aspect of Jacquline Catanazaro's respiratory difficulties, what mechanism(s) would you expect to be working to compensate for her respiratory acidosis?

7. If the client had electrolyte results available, what potential imbalances might you expect to find? Explain your answer. (*Hint:* See page 175 in your textbook.)

8. Based on Jacquline Catanazaro's medical diagnosis, what is the underlying pathophysiologic problem leading to the respiratory acidosis? (*Hint:* See page 1570 of the textbook.)

 • Click on **Return to Room 402**.
• Click on **Patient Care** and then **Physical Assessment**.

9. Perform a complete physical assessment on Jacquline Catanazaro and record your findings in the table below.

Areas Assessed	Findings on Physical Examination
Neurologic	
Musculoskeletal	
Cardiovascular	
Respiratory	
Integumentary	

10. Are there any clinical manifestations of respiratory acidosis? If so, please describe. If not, how do you explain this?

11. If Jacquline Catanazaro had a pH level of 7.2, how might this assessment differ?

- Click on **Chart** and then on **402**.
- Click on **Physician's Orders**.

12. Look at the most recent physician's orders. What medication is ordered to treat the client's respiratory acidosis? What is the medication's underlying mechanism of action to correct the acidosis?

Now let's check on this same client later in the day.

- Click on **Return to Room 402**.
- Click on **Leave the Floor** and then **Restart the Program**.
- Log in to Period of Care 2 and select Jacquline Catanazaro from the Patient List.
- Click on **Go to Nurses' Station**.
- Click on **Chart** and then on **402**.
- Click on **Laboratory Reports**.

13. Interpret the ABGs drawn at 1000. Was the treatment effective?

Clients Having Surgery

👓 **Reading Assignment:** Clients Having Surgery: Promoting Positive Outcomes
(Chapter 14)

Patient: Piya Jordan, Room 403

Goal: Use the nursing process to competently care for perioperative clients.

Objectives:

1. Document a complete history and physical on a preoperative client.
2. Identify appropriate rationales for preoperative orders on an assigned client.
3. Evaluate completeness of preoperative teaching on a client scheduled for surgery.
4. Document a focused assessment on a client transferred from PACU to a medical-surgical unit.
5. Plan appropriate interventions to prevent postoperative complications in an assigned client.
6. Use the nursing process to correctly administer scheduled and prn medications to an assigned client.

Overview:

In this lesson you will learn the essentials of caring for a client in both the preoperative and postoperative stages of surgery. You will document assessments, plan, implement, and evaluate care given. Piya Jordan is a 68-year-old female admitted after experiencing nausea and vomiting for 3 days. Begin this lesson by answering the following questions regarding concepts related to the care of surgical clients.

Exercise 1

 Clinical Preparation: Writing Activity

 10 minutes

1. Define or describe the following terms.

   a. Preoperative period:

   b. Intraoperative period:

   c. Postoperative period:

   d. Perioperative period:

   e. Perioperative nurse:

2. Identify three goals of perioperative nursing.

Exercise 2

 CD-ROM Activity

 40 minutes

- Sign in to work at Pacific View Regional Hospital for Period of Care 1. (*Note:* If you are already in the virtual hospital from a previous exercise, click on **Leave the Floor** and then **Restart the Program** to get to the sign-in window.)
- From the Patient List, select Piya Jordan (Room 403).
- Click on **Go to Nurses' Station**.
- Click on **Chart** and then on **403**.
- Click on **Emergency Department** and review this record.

1. What day and time did Piya Jordan arrive in the Emergency Department?

2. What complaints (problems) brought her to the ED?

3. What were Piya Jordan's primary and secondary admitting diagnoses?

 • Click on **Nursing Admission**.

 4. Important areas of data collection for the health history during the preoperative period are listed in the table below and on the next page. Using the Nursing Admission form as your source, record the data collected from Piya Jordan for each area. If an area was not completed, write "No data" in that section. (*Hint:* Refer to pages 184-186 of your textbook for clarification of each section.)

Areas of Data Collection	Piya Jordan's Data
Previous surgery and experience with anesthesia	

Areas of Data Collection	Piya Jordan's Data
Serious illness or trauma (ABCDE mnemonic)	
Alcohol, recreational drug, or nicotine use	
Current discomforts	
Chronic illnesses	
Advanced age	
Medication history	
Psychologic history	
Ability to tolerate perioperative stress	
Lifestyle habits	
Social history	

→ • Click on **History and Physical**.

5. In addition to data obtained from the health history and recorded in the Nursing Admission, a physical exam provides necessary data for the preoperative assessment. For each of the areas listed in the table below, identify (in the middle column) the key items to assess according to your textbook (pages 187-189). In the last column, document the results from the physician's assessment as noted in the History and Physical. If an area was not completed, write "No data" in that section. (*Note:* Do not include diagnostic testing—that will be addressed separately.)

Physical Examination Area	Key Specific Assessments from the Textbook	H&P Results for Piya Jordan
Cardiovascular		
Respiratory		
Musculoskeletal		
Gastrointestinal		
Skin integrity		
Renal		
Cognitive and neurologic		

➡ • Click on **Laboratory Reports**.

6. Common preoperative lab tests are listed in the table below. For each test, record the results for Piya Jordan. If a test was not completed, write "No data."

Laboratory Tests	Piya Jordan's Results
Potassium	
Sodium	
Chloride	
Calcium	
Magnesium	
Glucose (fasting)	
Carbon dioxide	
Creatinine	
BUN	
Albumin	
Prealbumin	
Hemoglobin	
Hematocrit	
WBC	
Differential count	
Segmented neutrophils	
Banded neutrophils	
Eosinophils	
Basophils	
Lymphocytes	
Monocytes	
PT	
aPTT	

• Click on **Diagnostic Reports**.

7. Other common diagnostic tests are listed below. For each test, record the results for Piya Jordan. If the test was not completed, write "No data."

Diagnostic Test	Results for Piya Jordan
ECG	
Chest x-ray	

8. Are any of Piya Jordan's lab and diagnostic results abnormal or of concern for a client preparing to undergo surgery? Explain.

 9. Based on your findings during this exercise, how would you rate Piya Jordan's general surgical risk according to the American Society of Anesthesiologists? (*Hint:* See Box 14-2 in your textbook.)

Exercise 3

 CD-ROM Activity

 30 minutes

- Sign in to work at Pacific View Regional Hospital for Period of Care 1. (*Note:* If you are already in the virtual hospital from a previous exercise, click on **Leave the Floor** and then **Restart the Program** to get to the sign-in window.)
- From the Patient List, select Piya Jordan (Room 403).
- Click on **Go to Nurses' Station**.
- Click on **Chart** and then on **403**.
- Click on **Consents**.

1. For what procedure(s) has Piya Jordan given written consent?

2. Who signed the consent form as the witness?

3. Who is responsible for providing detailed information about the procedure(s) for which Piya Jordan has given consent?

4. What is the nurse's responsibility in regard to obtaining informed consent?

→ • Click on **Physician's Orders**.

5. Look at the orders for Tuesday 0130. What consent was ordered by the physician?

6. By when does this consent need to be obtained?

7. What is the purpose for the mineral oil enema that was ordered to be given to Piya Jordan?

8. What diet has the physician ordered preoperatively? What is the purpose for this diet order?

9. What is the rationale for giving Piya Jordan a unit of fresh frozen plasma preoperatively? (*Hint:* See Physician's Progress Notes for Tuesday 0130.)

10. What is the rationale for ordering a dose of cefotetan on call to the OR? Is this a safe order to administer to Piya Jordan? Explain why or why not.

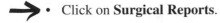 • Click on **Surgical Reports**.

11. Scroll down to the Preoperative Checklist. What preoperative teaching was completed?

12. The word *routines* on the preoperative checklist is not very specific. Explain specific items that should have been taught to Piya Jordan preoperatively.

LESSON 7

Cancer

⟋ᴏⳆᴏ **Reading Assignment:** Perspectives in Oncology (Chapter 16)
Clients with Cancer (Chapter 17)

Patient: Pablo Rodriguez, Room 405

Goal: Use the nursing process to competently care for clients with cancer.

Objectives:

1. Describe clinical manifestations and treatment for a client with cancer.
2. Recognize special needs of clients undergoing treatment for cancer.
3. Appropriately treat a client's symptoms related to disease process and/or side effects of treatment.
4. Discuss medications prescribed for a client with cancer, including expected therapeutic effects as well as adverse/side effects to monitor for.
5. Plan appropriate general interventions to prevent and/or treat complications related to chemotherapy.

Overview:

In this lesson you will learn the essentials of caring for a client diagnosed with cancer. You will collect data, assess, plan, implement, and evaluate care given. Pablo Rodriguez is a 71-year-old male admitted with advanced lung carcinoma. Begin this lesson by reviewing the general concepts of cancer as presented in your textbook.

Exercise 1

 Clinical Preparation: Writing Activity

 15 minutes

1. Identify and briefly describe four types of carcinogens.

2. What are the three types of therapies used to treat cancer? Describe their respective mechanisms of action.

3. List common side effects of chemotherapy.

4. What are some common side effects associated with radiation therapy (XRT)?

 5. List the warning signals associated with lung cancer. (*Hint:* See Box 62-3 in your textbook.)

Exercise 2

 CD-ROM Activity

 30 minutes

- Sign in to work at Pacific View Regional Hospital for Period of Care 1. (*Note:* If you are already in the virtual hospital from a previous exercise, click on **Leave the Floor** and then **Restart the Program** to get to the sign-in window.)
- From the Patient List, select Pablo Rodriguez (Room 405).
- Click on **Go to Nurses' Station**.
- Click on **Chart** and then on **405**.
- Click on **History and Physical**.

1. What is Pablo Rodriguez's main diagnosis?

2. How long ago was he diagnosed?

3. What risk factor for lung cancer is documented on the H&P?

4. What are other risk factors for lung cancer?

5. What clinical manifestations documented in the physician's review of systems are related to this disease process?

6. What treatment has Pablo Rodriguez received so far?

7. How long ago did Pablo Rodriguez receive his last chemotherapy?

8. What are the mechanism of action and the major side effects of docetaxel?

9. What is the nadir (the point at which the drug has the greatest impact on the bone marrow) of docetaxel? Would the client still be having side effects from this drug? Why or why not?

10. What interventions would you teach Pablo Rodriguez to prevent complications related to bone marrow suppression caused by chemotherapy?

Exercise 3

 CD-ROM Activity

 30 minutes

- Sign in to work at Pacific View Regional Hospital for Period of Care 2. (*Note:* If you are already in the virtual hospital from a previous exercise, click on **Leave the Floor** and then **Restart the Program** to get to the sign-in window.)
- From the Patient List, select Pablo Rodriguez (Room 405).
- Click on **Get Report** and read the change-of-shift report.

1. What unresolved problem for Pablo Rodriguez is noted in the change-of-shift report?

- Click on **Go to Nurses' Station**.
- Click on **Chart** and then on **405**.
- Click on **Nurse's Notes**.

2. Look at the note for Wednesday at 0415. How did the nurse respond to Pablo Rodriguez's complaints? Were the nurse's actions appropriate? Explain.

3. How might you have responded differently?

 • Click on **Return to Nurses' Station**.
 • Click on **405** to go to the client's room.
 • Click on **Patient Care** and then on **Nurse-Client Interactions**.
 • Select and view the video titled **0735: Patient Perceptions**. (*Note:* Check the virtual clock to see whether enough time has elapsed. You can use the fast-forward feature to advance the time by 2-minute intervals if the video is not yet available. Then click again on **Patient Care** and **Nurse-Client Interactions** to refresh the screen.)

4. What are Pablo Rodriguez's two major concerns at this point?

5. What other assessment should you perform before treating his complaint of nausea?

 • Click on **MAR**.
 • Click on tab **405** for Pablo Rodriguez's record.

6. What is ordered to manage the client's pain and nausea?

7. What might the nurse question regarding these medication orders?

- Click on **Return to Room 405**.
- Click on **Chart** and then on **405**.
- Click on **Nursing Admission**.

8. What is the client's weight in lb? In kg?

- Click on **Return to Room 405**.
- Click on the **Drug** icon in the lower left corner of your screen.

9. Calculate the maximum 24-hour dose for clients receiving the drug ordered for nausea (the drug you identified in question 6).

10. Calculate the maximum 24-hour dose for clients receiving this drug for management of postoperative nausea and vomiting.

11. Calculate the maximum amount of this drug Pablo Rodriguez could receive per 24 hours as ordered. Is it within the dosage guidelines? Is there any reason to be concerned about this dosage schedule over long periods of time?

12. What are the possible ramifications of giving high doses of this drug?

13. What are the ramifications of *not* giving this drug for the client's complaint of nausea?

14. If the nurse administers the prn Reglan at 0730, what should be done with the regularly scheduled 0800 dose?

LESSON **8**

Pain

/OZD **Reading Assignment:** Clients with Pain (Chapter 20)

Patients: Clarence Hughes, Room 404
Pablo Rodriguez, Room 405

Goal: Demonstrate understanding and application of appropriate interventions when caring for clients with pain.

Objectives:

1. Define the concept of pain.
2. Describe the source and type of pain for each assigned client.
3. Perform a comprehensive pain assessment for each client.
4. Identify variables that influence each client's perception of pain.
5. Safely administer analgesic medications to a client experiencing pain.
6. Plan appropriate nonpharmacologic measures that may be used to treat each client's pain.

Overview:

In this lesson you will evaluate the pain experiences of two different clients—from assessment to management. Clarence Hughes is a 73-year-old male who is status post total knee arthroplasty. Pablo Rodriguez is a 71-year-old male admitted with advanced lung carcinoma. Begin this activity by reviewing the general concepts presented in your textbook. Answer the following questions to solidify your understanding of pain.

Exercise 1

 Clinical Preparation: Writing Activity

 15 minutes

1. Using the definitions of pain provided in the textbook, describe pain in your own words.

2. Define the following terms related to pain.

   a. Nociceptor

   b. Nociception

   c. Hyperalgesia

   d. Breakthrough pain

   e. Psychogenic pain

3. What is the difference between a client's pain threshold and pain tolerance?

4. Various organizations have developed guidelines for pain management. What are the five common elements contained in all these?

Exercise 2

 CD-ROM Activity

 45 minutes

- Sign in to work at Pacific View Regional Hospital for Period of Care 1. (*Note:* If you are already in the virtual hospital from a previous exercise, click on **Leave the Floor** and then **Restart the Program** to get to the sign-in window.)
- From the Patient List, select Clarence Hughes (Room 404).
- Click on **Get Report**.

1. What information is obtained during report concerning Clarence Hughes' most recent pain assessment?

Now complete your own pain assessment on Clarence Hughes.

 • Click on **Go to Nurses' Station**.
- Click on **404** to go to the patient's room.
- Inside the room, click on **Take Vital Signs**.

2. How does Clarence Hughes rate his pain at the present time?

 • Click on **Patient Care** and then **Physical Assessment**.
- Select the various body area buttons and assessment subcategories as needed to answer question 3.

3. Perform a focused assessment on Clarence Hughes. Record your findings below.

 • Click on **Patient Care** and then **Nurse-Client Interactions**.

• Select and view the video titled **0730: Assessment/Perception of Care**. (*Note:* Check the virtual clock to see whether enough time has elapsed. You can use the fast-forward feature to advance the time by 2-minute intervals if the video is not yet available. Then click again on **Patient Care** and **Nurse-Client Interactions** to refresh the screen.)

4. How does Clarence Hughes describe his pain? Describe his nonverbal communication. Do his nonverbal cues correlate with his complaint of pain?

5. The nurse asks Clarence Hughes if she may perform an assessment prior to medicating him for pain. Is this appropriate? Why or why not?

• Click on **EPR** and then on **Login**.

• Select **404** as the Patient and **Vital Signs** as the Category.

6. Document Clarence Hughes' pain rating and characteristics over the last 24 hours in the table below and on the next page. (*Note:* You will complete the final column in question 7.)

Time of Assessment	Pain Rating	Pain Characteristic	Name of Analgesic Administered
Tuesday 0700			
Tuesday 0815			
Tuesday 0930			

Time of Assessment	Pain Rating	Pain Characteristic	Name of Analgesic Administered
Tuesday 1230			
Tuesday 1330			
Tuesday 1500			
Tuesday 1630			
Tuesday 1700			
Tuesday 2030			
Tuesday 2300			
Wednesday 0200			
Wednesday 0715			

- Click on **Exit EPR**.
- Click on **Chart** and then on **404**.
- Click on **Expired MARs**.

7. Review the expired MARs to note the times of analgesic administration for Clarence Hughes. Document your findings in the far right column of the table in question 6.

- Click on **Return to Room 404**.
- Click on **Kardex** and then on tab **404**.

8. What is the stated outcome related to comfort for Clarence Hughes? Is this a measurable outcome? How might you improve the writing of the outcome?

9. Based on the stated outcome, review the table you completed for questions 6 and 7. Was the administered pain medication effective? Give a rationale for your answer.

10. Was the client's pain assessed appropriately following each analgesic administration? Explain your answer.

11. What is the physiologic source of Clarence Hughes' pain? What type of pain is he experiencing? Explain your answer. (*Hint:* See pages 353-354 of your textbook.)

12. Is the ordered analgesic medication appropriate for this type of pain? If not, what would you suggest? Are there any nonpharmacologic interventions that might be helpful for Clarence Hughes? Explain your answer.

13. What nursing assessments should be completed before administration of oxycodone with acetaminophen?

14. For what common side effects should the nurse monitor Clarence Hughes related to opioid use? (*Hint:* If you need help, return to the Nurses' Station and click on the Drug Guide on the counter or on the **Drug** icon in the lower left corner of your screen.)

→ • Click on **Return to Room 404**.
   • Click on **Chart** and then **404**.
   • Click on **Nurse's Notes**.

15. According to the note for Wednesday at 0715, which of the side effects identified in question 14 is Clarence Hughes experiencing? What should the nurse do to treat and/or prevent this side effect?

Since Clarence Hughes received his last dose of pain medication at 0200, it is now appropriate to administer another dose. Prepare to administer a dose of analgesic to Clarence Hughes by completing the following steps:

Medication Preparation

- Click on **Return to Room 404** and then **Nurses' Station**.
- Click on **Medication Room** on the bottom of your screen.
- Access the Automated System by either selecting the icon at the top of the screen or by clicking on the **Automated System** cart in center of screen.
- Click on **Login**.
- Choose Clarence Hughes in box 1 and Automated System Drawer (G-O) in box 2. Click **Open Drawer** and review the list of available medications. (*Note:* You may click **Review MAR** at any time to verify correct medication order. Remember to look at patient name on MAR to make sure you have the correct MAR—you must click on the correct room number within the MAR. Click on **Return to Medication Room** after reviewing the correct MAR.)
- From the Open Drawer view, select the correct medication to administer. Click **Put Medication on Tray** and then click **Close Drawer**.
- Click on **View Medication Room**.
- Begin the preparation process by clicking **Preparation** at the top of screen or clicking on the tray on the counter on the left side of the Medication Room.
- Click **Prepare**, fill in any requested data in the Preparation Wizard, and click **Next**. Then select the correct patient and click on **Finish**.
- You can click on **Review Your Medications** and then on **Return to Medication Room** when ready. Once you are back in the Medication Room, you may go directly to Clarence Hughes' room to administer this medication by clicking on **404** at the bottom of the screen.

Medication Administration

- Administer the medication utilizing the five rights of medication administration. After you have collected the appropriate assessment data and are ready for administration, click **Patient Care** and then **Medication Administration**. Verify that the correct patient and medication(s) appear in the left-hand window. Then click the down arrow next to Select. From the drop-down menu, select **Administer** and complete the Administration Wizard by providing any information requested. When the Wizard stops asking for information, click **Administer to Patient**. Specify **Yes** when asked whether this administration should be recorded in the MAR. Finally, click **Finish**.

Now let's see how you did!

- Click on **Leave the Floor** at the bottom of your screen. From the Floor Menu, select **Look at Your Preceptor's Evaluation**. Then click on **Medication Scorecard** in Clarence Hughes' box.

16. Disregard the report for the routine scheduled medications but note whether or not you correctly administered the analgesic medication. If not, why do you think you were incorrect in administering this drug? According to Table C in this scorecard, what are the appropriate resources that should be used prior to administering this medication? Did you use them correctly?

Exercise 3

 CD-ROM Activity

 45 minutes

- Sign in to work at Pacific View Regional Hospital for Period of Care 1. (*Note:* If you are already in the virtual hospital from a previous exercise, click on **Leave the Floor** and then **Restart the Program** to get to the sign-in window.)
- From the Patient List, select Pablo Rodriguez (Room 405).
- Click on **Get Report**.

1. What information is obtained during report concerning Pablo Rodriguez's most recent pain assessment?

Now complete your own pain assessment of Pablo Rodriguez.

 • Click on **Go to Nurses' Station**.
- Click on **405**.
- Click on **Take Vital Signs**.

2. How does Pablo Rodriguez rate his pain at the present time?

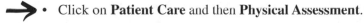 • Click on **Patient Care** and then **Physical Assessment**.

3. Perform a focused assessment on Pablo Rodriguez. Document your findings below.

 • Click on **Chart** and then **405**.
- Click on **Nursing Admission**.

4. Scroll down to page 22 of the Nursing Admission form. What are the aggravating and alleviating factors related to Pablo Rodriguez's pain?

 • Click on **Return to Room 405** and then on **Patient Care**.
• Click on **Nurse-Client Interactions**.
• Select and view the video titled **0730: Symptom Management**. (*Note:* Check the virtual clock to see whether enough time has elapsed. You can use the fast-forward feature to advance the time by 2-minute intervals if the video is not yet available. Then click again on **Patient Care** and **Nurse-Client Interactions** to refresh the screen.)

5. What sociocultural influences are affecting Pablo Rodriguez's perception and management of pain?

 • Click on **EPR** and then on **Login**.
• Select **405** as the Patient and **Vital Signs** as the Category.

6. In the table below, document Pablo Rodriguez's pain rating and characteristics since admission (columns 2 and 3). (*Note:* You will complete this table in question 7.)

Time of Assessment	Pain Rating	Pain Characteristic	Time of Medication Administration	Name and Dose of Analgesic Administered
Tuesday 2300				
			Wednesday 0100	
Wednesday 0300				
Wednesday 0700			Wednesday 0700	

→ • Click on **Exit EPR**.
  • Click on **Chart** and then on **405**.
  • Click on **Expired MARs**.

7. Review the expired MARs to find the times of analgesic administration for Pablo Rodriguez. Document your findings in the far right column of the table in question 6.

→ • Click on **Return to Room 405**.
  • Click on **Kardex**.
  • Click on tab **405** for the correct record.

8. What is the stated outcome related to comfort for Pablo Rodriguez? Is this a measurable outcome? How might you improve the writing of the outcome?

9. Based on the stated outcome, review the table you completed for questions 6 and 7, as well as your pain assessment in question 2. Was the administered pain medication effective? Give a rationale for your answer.

10. Was the client's pain assessed appropriately following each analgesic administration? Explain your answer.

11. What is the physiologic source of Pablo Rodriguez's pain? What type of pain is he experiencing? Explain your answer. (*Hint:* See pages 353-354 of your textbook.)

12. Is the ordered analgesic medication appropriate for this type of pain? If not, what would you suggest? Are there any nonpharmacologic interventions that might be helpful for Pablo Rodriguez? Explain your answer.

 • Click on **Return to Room 405**.
   • Click on **Patient Care** and then **Nurse-Client Interactions**.
   • Select and view the video titled **0735: Patient Perceptions**. (*Note:* Check the virtual clock to see whether enough time has elapsed. You can use the fast-forward feature to advance the time by 2-minute intervals if the video is not yet available. Then click again on **Patient Care** and **Nurse-Client Interactions** to refresh the screen.)

13. Discuss the nurse's evaluation of Pablo Rodriguez's understanding and use of the PCA pump. Do you think the nurse's actions are therapeutic? If not, what other approaches would you suggest?

14. What nursing assessments and interventions are appropriate for clients receiving IV morphine sulfate? (*Note:* For help, return to the **Nurses' Station** and click on the Drug Guide on the counter or click on the **Drug** icon in the lower left corner of your screen.)

9

Palliative Care

 Reading Assignment: Perspectives in Palliative Care (Chapter 21)

Patient: Pablo Rodriguez, Room 405

Goal: Demonstrate understanding and appropriate application of palliative care concepts.

Objectives:

1. Identify appropriate application of palliative care concepts for a client with a terminal illness.
2. Assess and identify common distressing symptoms present in a terminally ill client.
3. Choose interventions appropriate to relieve distressing symptoms in a terminally ill client.
4. Describe appropriate communication techniques when dealing with a terminally ill client and family.

Overview:

In this lesson you will describe, plan, and evaluate the care of a client with a terminal illness that is no longer responding to therapy. Pablo Rodriguez is a 71-year-old male suffering from advanced lung carcinoma, diagnosed 1 year ago.

Exercise 1

Clinical Preparation: Writing Activity

10 minutes

1. Define *palliative care*.

2. What are the two major goals of palliative care?

3. Identify seven symptoms at the end of life that a palliative plan of care would address.

Exercise 2

 CD-ROM Activity

 30 minutes

*   Sign in to work at Pacific View Regional Hospital for Period of Care 3. (*Note:* If you are already in the virtual hospital from a previous exercise, click on **Leave the Floor** and then **Restart the Program** to get to the sign-in window.)
*   From the Patient List, select Pablo Rodriguez (Room 405).
*   Click on **Go to Nurses' Station**.
*   Click on **Chart** and then on **405**.
*   Click on **Emergency Department**.

1. Why was Pablo Rodriguez admitted to the hospital?

2. What are his primary and secondary diagnoses?

➤ • Click on **Nursing Admission**.

3. What does the admitting nurse document for this client's anticipated needs for support at time of discharge?

4. What documentation in the Nursing Admission would support the presence of cachexia in Pablo Rodriguez?

5. What collaborative interventions would be appropriate to address Pablo Rodriguez's nutritional problems?

6. What distressing symptoms are noted in the Activity/Rest section of the Nursing Admission form?

7. What interventions would you plan for Pablo Rodriguez in order to alleviate these concerns?

• Click on **Return to Nurses' Station** and then on **405**.

- Click on **Patient Care** and then **Nurse-Client Interactions**.
- Select and view the video titled **1530: Decision—End-of-Life Care**. (*Note:* Check the virtual clock to see whether enough time has elapsed. You can use the fast-forward feature to advance the time by 2-minute intervals if the video is not yet available. Then click again on **Patient Care** and **Nurse-Client Interactions** to refresh the screen.)

8. What is Pablo Rodriguez telling the nurse?

9. What therapeutic communication techniques is the nurse using? Are they effective? What other technique(s) might have been used?

 10. Although Pablo Rodriguez's family is not currently present, how might the nurse plan to help the family meet the client's physical and emotional needs when he goes home? (*Hint:* See Table 21-7 in the textbook.)

Exercise 3

  CD-ROM Activity

45 minutes

- Sign in to work at Pacific View Regional Hospital for Period of Care 1. (*Note:* If you are already in the virtual hospital from a previous exercise, click on **Leave the Floor** and then **Restart the Program** to get to the sign-in window.)
- From the Patient List, select Pablo Rodriguez (Room 405).
- Click on **Go to Nurses' Station**.
- Click on **405** to go to the patient's room.
- Read the **Initial Observations** at 0730.

1. According to the Initial Observations, what physical symptom of distress is Pablo Rodriguez displaying?

2. How would you intervene to alleviate Pablo Rodriguez's symptoms? Provide rationales for your interventions. (*Hint:* You may need to go to the client's chart to review the physician's orders.)

 • Click on **EPR** and then **Login**.
- Select **405** as the Patient and **Vital Signs** as the Category.
- Look at the vital sign assessment documented on Wednesday at 0700.

3. Describe Pablo Rodriguez's pain assessment.

4. What interventions would be appropriate to relieve this pain?

Now let's check the client's current vital signs.

➡ • Click on **Exit EPR**.
   • Click on **Take Vital Signs**. (*Note:* Pain assessment is now considered the fifth vital sign.)

   5. Based on the EPR data and Pablo Rodriguez's current pain rating, is the morphine providing effective relief? Explain.

➡ • Click on **Patient Care** and then **Physcial Assessment**.
   • From the list of body areas (the yellow buttons), click on **Abdomen**.
   • From the system subcategories, click on **Gastrointestinal**.

   6. Document your GI assessment findings below. What is this significance of these findings? How do they relate to Pablo Rodriguez's diagnosis and/or treatment?

   7. How would you intervene to prevent potential complications related to the above findings?

• Click on **Patient Care** and then **Nurse-Client Interactions**.

- Select and view the video titled **0730: Symptom Management**. (*Note:* Check the virtual clock to see whether enough time has elapsed. You can use the fast-forward feature to advance the time by 2-minute intervals if the video is not yet available. Then click again on **Patient Care** and **Nurse-Client Interactions** to refresh the screen.)

8. Describe Pablo Rodriguez's emotional distress as displayed in this video.

9. What nursing interventions would be appropriate to help Pablo Rodriguez cope?

- Now select and view the video titled **0735: Patient Perceptions**. (*Note:* Check the virtual clock to see whether enough time has elapsed. You can use the fast-forward feature to advance the time by 2-minute intervals if the video is not yet available. Then click again on **Patient Care** and **Nurse-Client Interactions** to refresh the screen.)

10. Now that his pain is controlled, what does Pablo Rodriguez complain of (in addition to not being able to rest)? How would you intervene to relieve this additional discomfort?

11. Recall the definition you provided of *palliative care* earlier in this lesson. Based on your observations during this exercise, do you believe Pablo Rodriguez is receiving such care? Why or why not?

Substance Abuse

 Reading Assignment: Clients with Substance Abuse Disorders (Chapter 24)

Patient: Harry George, Room 401

Goal: Demonstrate understanding and appropriate application of nursing interventions for clients with substance abuse disorders.

Objectives:

1. Identify risk factors associated with substance abuse.
2. Describe assessment findings related to the use and abuse of nicotine and alcohol.
3. Describe assessment findings related to withdrawal from nicotine and alcohol.
4. Examine alcohol withdrawal protocols for the care of a client admitted to an acute care setting.
5. Identify appropriate nursing interventions when caring for a client with a substance abuse disorder.

Overview:

In this lesson you will learn about the care of a client undergoing specific substance abuse issues. Harry George is a 54-year-old male admitted with infection and swelling of his left foot and a history of type 2 diabetes. Begin this activity by reviewing the general concepts presented in your textbook. Answer the following questions to solidify your understanding of substance abuse.

Exercise 1

Clinical Preparation: Writing Activity

5 minutes

1. Define *substance abuse*.

2. What is the difference between physiologic and psychologic dependence?

3. Define the term *addiction*.

Exercise 2

 CD-ROM Activity

 30 minutes

- Sign in to work at Pacific View Regional Hospital for Period of Care 1. (*Note:* If you are already in the virtual hospital from a previous exercise, click on **Leave the Floor** and then **Restart the Program** to get to the sign-in window.)
- From the Patient List, select Harry George (Room 401).
- Click on **Go to Nurses' Station**.
- Click on **Chart** and then on **401**.
- Click on **Emergency Department** and read this record.

1. What are Harry George's primary and secondary diagnoses?

2. What specific risk factors for alcoholism are noted in the Emergency Department Record? (*Hint:* Read the admitting physician notes.) Describe how the risk factors contribute to alcohol abuse.

3. When did Harry George begin drinking excessively? Was there a precipitating event that contributed to this problem?

4. What other documentation is found in the Emergency Department Record to support the diagnosis of alcohol abuse?

5. Is there any evidence of nicotine addiction?

→ • Click on **History and Physical**.

6. Read the Physical Examination report on page 4 of the H&P. What assessment findings may be related to Harry George's alcohol abuse?

7. What further history is obtained regarding nicotine abuse?

8. What physical examination finding(s) may be related to cigarette smoking?

• Click on **Laboratory Reports**.

9. What was Harry George's blood alcohol level on admission?

10. What clinical manifestations would you expect to find based on this level?

 • Click on **Return to Nurses' Station**.
   • Click on **401** to go to Harry George's room.
   • Click on **Patient Care** and then **Nurse-Client Interactions**.
   • Select and view the video titled **0735: Symptom Management**. (*Note:* Check the virtual clock to see whether enough time has elapsed. You can use the fast-forward feature to advance the time by 2-minute intervals if the video is not yet available. Then click again on **Patient Care** and **Nurse-Client Interactions** to refresh the screen.)

11. What visual assessment findings noted on this video might suggest withdrawal symptoms for Harry George?

Exercise 3

  CD-ROM Activity

45 minutes

- Sign in to work at Pacific View Regional Hospital for Period of Care 4. (*Note:* If you are already in the virtual hospital from a previous exercise, click on **Leave the Floor** and then **Restart the Program** to get to the sign-in window.)
- Click on **Chart** and then on **401**. (*Remember:* You are not able to visit patients or administer medications during Period of Care 4. You are able to review patients' records only.)
- Click on **Mental Health**.

1. Read the Psychiatric/Mental Health Assessment for Harry George. What risk factors for substance abuse are noted on this assessment?

→ • Click on **Nurse's Notes**.

2. How does the nurse describe Harry George's behavior now?

3. The textbook identifies the following symptoms of clients in alcohol withdrawal. Put an X next to each symptom that applies for Harry George. Select all that apply.

_____ a. Tremors

_____ b. Weakness

_____ c. Nausea

_____ d. Vomiting

_____ e. Sweating

_____ f. Tachycardia

_____ g. Hypertension

_____ h. Agitated behavior

_____ i. Delusions

_____ j. Hallucinations and nocturnal illusions

→ • Click on **Emergency Department**.

4. At what time did Harry George have his last alcoholic drink? Calculate the number of hours that have passed since his last drink and compare this with the usual time frame noted for withdrawal symptoms.

→ • Click on **History and Physical**.

5. At the end of the H&P, the physician writes a plan of care. What pharmacologic interventions is the physician planning to prevent and/or treat alcohol withdrawal?

6. What is the intended benefit of thiamine administration for this client? (*Hint:* For help, return to the Nurses' Station and click on the Drug Guide on the counter or click on the **Drug** icon in the lower left corner of your screen.)

7. What is the classification of chlordiazepoxide? Identify this drug's most common brand name. What is the intended therapeutic effect of this drug for Harry George?

8. What are the advantages of using medications in the above classification over other types of medications? (*Hint:* See pages 438-439 of your textbook.)

➤ • Click on **Nurse's Notes**. (*Note:* If you are currently within the Drug Guide, first click **Return to Nurses' Station**; then click on **Chart**, on **401**, and on **Nurses' Notes**.)

9. Read the notes dated Wednesday at 1245 and again at 1315. Is the chlordiazepoxide effective? Explain your answer.

10. What is the classification of lorazepam? Identify this drug's most common brand name. What is the intended therapeutic effect of this drug for Harry George?

11. Are there any potential drug interactions between chlordiazepoxide and lorazepam? If so, please elaborate.

12. Since both Librium and Ativan are ordered for similar therapeutic effects, what factors would influence the nurse's decision regarding which medication to use? (*Hint:* Consult the MAR.)

➤ • Click on **Physician's Orders**.

13. What is the most recent physician order?

→ • Click on **Physician's Notes**.

14. Read the most recent physician's progress note. What is the rationale for writing the order you identified in question 13?

15. Based on your readings in the textbook (pages 438-439), what interventions would you expect to be part of an alcohol withdrawal protocol?

→ • Click on **Nurse's Notes**.

16. Read the note for Wednesday at 1800. What clinical manifestations of nicotine withdrawal is the client exhibiting?

17. According to your textbook, after how many hours of abstinence do nicotine withdrawal symptoms begin to appear?

18. How long has Harry George been without cigarettes? (*Hint:* Look at time and date of the first Nurse's Note.)

 19. What is the effect of simultaneous alcohol and nicotine withdrawal? (Hint: See Box 24-5 in your textbook.)

20. What typical manifestations of nicotine withdrawal might be found i a different client who was withdrawing *only* from nicotine?

21. To plan nursing care for Harry George, identify three priority nursing diagnoses for the client problems listed in the following table. For each diagnosis, identify related client outcomes and appropriate nursing interventions to achieve these outcomes.

Client Problems (Assessment)	Nursing Diagnosis	Goals/Outcomes (Planning)	Nursing Interventions
Tremors			
Anxiety			
Malnutrition			

LESSON **11** _____

Osteoarthritis and Total Knee Replacement

_____

/CD **Reading Assignment:** Management of Clients with Musculoskeletal Disorders
(Chapter 26)

Patient: Clarence Hughes, Room 404

Goal: Use the nursing process to competently care for clients with musculoskeletal disorders.

Objectives:

1. Describe clinical manifestations and treatment for a client with debilitating osteoarthritis.
2. Document a focused assessment on a postoperative client who has undergone a total knee arthroplasty.
3. Plan appropriate interventions to prevent complications related to a total knee replacement in an assigned client.
4. Identify and provide rationale for collaborative care measures used to treat a client after a total knee arthroplasty.

Overview:

In this lesson you will learn the essentials of caring for a client undergoing a total knee arthroplasty for treatment of debilitating osteoarthritis. You will document, assess, plan, implement, and evaluate care given. Clarence Hughes is a 73-year-old male admitted for an elective knee replacement. Begin this lesson by reviewing the general concepts of acid-base balance as presented in your textbook.

Exercise 1

Clinical Preparation: Writing Activity

10 minutes

1. List risk factors related to the occurrence of idiopathic (primary) and secondary osteoarthritis (OA).

2. Briefly describe the general pathophysiology of OA.

3. What are the clinical manifestations of OA?

4. What laboratory and/or radiographic testing are used in the diagnosis of OA?

Exercise 2

  CD-ROM Activity

40 minutes

- Sign in to work at Pacific View Regional Hospital for Period of Care 1. (*Note:* If you are already in the virtual hospital from a previous exercise, click on **Leave the Floor** and then **Restart the Program** to get to the sign-in window.)
- From the Patient List, select Clarence Hughes (Room 404).
- Click on **Go to Nurses' Station**.
- Click on **Chart** and then on **404**.
- Click on **History and Physical**.

1. Why was Clarence Hughes admitted to the hospital?

2. Describe the symptoms that brought him to this point.

3. According to the H&P, what medications and/or treatments were used to treat Clarence Hughes before he elected to have surgery?

4. Explain the rationale for performing a total knee replacement on Clarence Hughes.

→ • Click on **Surgical Reports**.

5. How does the report of operation describe the surgical procedure performed on Clarence Hughes?

6. Based on your reading from the textbook, what can you add to the description of a total knee arthroplasty?

7. What medication was added to the cement used for this procedure? Explain the rationale for the use of this medication.

8. What was Clarence Hughes' estimated blood loss (EBL)?

- Click on **Physician's Orders**.
- Scroll down to read the orders for Sunday 1600.

9. What frequent assessments are ordered? Describe specifically how these assessments are completed and what the nurse is looking for.

10. What drain is ordered for Clarence Hughes? What is the expected amount of drainage?

- Click on **Return to Nurses' Station**.
- Click on **EPR** and then on **Login**.
- Select **404** as the Patient and **Intake and Output** as the Category.

11. Find "Output: Drain #1" for documentation of hemovac drainage. How much total drainage is recorded?

- Click on **Exit EPR**.
- Click on **Chart** and then **404**.
- Click on **Physician's Orders**.
- Find the orders for Monday 0715.

12. What is ordered for Clarence Hughes' left knee? Explain the purpose and basic use of this device.

 13. According to your textbook (page 486), what does evidence-based practice conclude regarding the use of the CPM machine?

14. How should Clarence Hughes' operative leg be positioned in bed when not using the CPM? Explain the rationale for this position.

→ • Click on **Laboratory Reports**.

15. What was Clarence Hughes' H&H on Tuesday at 0600?

16. Why do you think his H&H was decreased? (*Hint:* Check his admitting H&H, EBL, drainage output, and intravenous intake.)

→ • Click on **Physician's Orders**.

17. What was ordered to correct the above laboratory result?

Exercise 3

 CD-ROM Activity

 45 minutes

- Sign in to work at Pacific View Regional Hospital for Period of Care 1. (*Note:* If you are already in the virtual hospital from a previous exercise, click on **Leave the Floor** and then **Restart the Program** to get to the sign-in window.)
- From the Patient List, select Clarence Hughes (Room 404).
- Click on **Get Report**.

1. What are your concerns for Clarence Hughes after receiving report?

 • Click on **Go to Nurses' Station**.
- Click on **404** to go to Clarence Hughes' room.
- Click on **Patient Care** and then **Physical Assessment**.

2. Based on Clarence Hughes' diagnosis and surgery, complete a focused assessment and document your findings below and on the next page.

Area Assessed	Findings
Integumentary	
Musculoskeletal	
Neurovascular	

Area Assessed	Findings
Gastrointestinal	
Respiratory	

 • Click on **Clinical Alerts**.

3. Based on these findings, what would be your priority interventions?

Medication Preparation

 • Click on **Medication Room**.

• Click on **MAR** to determine prn medications that have been ordered for Clarence Hughes to address his constipation and pain. (*Note:* You may click on **Review MAR** at any time to verify correct medication order. Remember to look at the patient name on the MAR to make sure you have the correct patient's record; you must click on the correct room number within the MAR. Click on **Return to Medication Room** after reviewing the correct MAR.)

• Click on **Unit Dosage** (or on the Unit Dosage cabinet); from the close-up view, click on drawer **404**.

• Select the medications you would like to administer. After each selection, click **Put Medication on Tray**. When you are finished selecting medications, click **Close Drawer**.

• Click on **View Medication Room**.

• Click on **Automated System** (or on the Automated System unit itself). Click **Login**.

• On the next screen, specify the correct patient and drawer location.

• Select the medication you would like to administer and click on **Put Medication on Tray**. Repeat this process if you wish to administer other medications from the Automated System.

• When you are finished, click **Close Drawer**. At the bottom right corner of the next screen, click on **View Medication Room**.

• From the Medication Room, click on **Preparation** (or on the preparation tray).

• Click **Next**, specify the correct patient to administer this medication to, and click **Finish**.

• Repeat the previous two steps until all medications that you want to administer are prepared.

- You can click on **Review Your Medications** and then on **Return to Medication Room** when ready. Once you are back in the Medication Room, you may go directly to Clarence Hughes' room by clicking on **404** at the bottom of the screen.

Medication Administration

- Administer the medication(s), utilizing the five rights of medication administration. After you have collected the appropriate assessment data and are ready for administration, click **Patient Care** and then **Medication Administration**. Verify that the correct patient and medication(s) appear in the left-hand window. Then click the down arrow next to Select. From the drop-down menu, select **Administer** and complete the Administration Wizard by providing any information requested. When the Wizard stops asking for information, click **Administer to Patient**. Specify **Yes** when asked whether this administration should be recorded in the MAR. Finally, click **Finish**. You will evaluate your performance in this area at the end of this exercise (see question 14).

4. What is missing on the client's order for oxycodone with acetaminophen? What measures need to be taken?

5. Based on the knowledge that most antacids decrease absorption of other medications when concurrently administered, what options might the nurse employ to ensure adequate absorption of pain medication? (*Hint:* To consult the Drug Guide, return to the Nurses' Station and click on the Drug Guide on the counter or click on the **Drug** icon in the lower left corner of your screen.)

• Still in the patient's room, click on **Patient Care** and then **Nurse-Client Interactions**.

• Select and view the video titled **0735: Empathy**. (*Note:* Check the virtual clock to see whether enough time has elapsed. You can use the fast-forward feature to advance the time by 2-minute intervals if the video is not yet available. Then click again on **Patient Care** and **Nurse-Client Interactions** to refresh the screen.)

6. In the video, the nurse attempts to appear empathetic by offering to listen to the client's concerns. Are her actions congruent with her verbal communication? Why or why not?

7. What would you, as a student nurse, do differently?

8. Potential complications related to Clarence Hughes' postoperative status are listed below and on the next page. While planning nursing care for this client, identify measures that can be employed to prevent these complications. Document your plan of care below. (*Hint:* Postoperative care for a client with a TKA is similar to care for a client with a THA.)

Complications	Preventative Measures
Neurovascular compromise	
Wound infection	

Complications	Preventative Measures
Limited range of motion	
DVT	
Bleeding/anemia	

 • Click on **Chart** and then on **404**.
 • Click on **Consultations**.

9. What is physical therapy (PT) doing for Clarence Hughes?

 • Click on **Physician's Orders**.

10. What is the client's activity order for Wednesday morning?

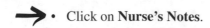 • Click on **Nurse's Notes**.

11. What is the client's goal for CPM therapy today?

12. Do you think the ambulation and CPM goals are sufficient for the client to be discharged tomorrow? Why or why not? (*Hint:* Review his home situation in the Nursing Admission form.)

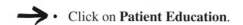 • Click on **Patient Education**.

13. What teaching should be completed for Clarence Hughes prior to discharge?

Now let's see how you did with the medication administration!

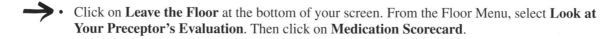 • Click on **Leave the Floor** at the bottom of your screen. From the Floor Menu, select **Look at Your Preceptor's Evaluation**. Then click on **Medication Scorecard**.

14. Ignore the information for giving regularly scheduled medications. Note whether or not you correctly administered the appropriate prn medications. If not, why do you think you were incorrect? According to Table C in this scorecard, what are the appropriate resources that should be used and important assessments that should be completed before administering these medications? Did you use these resources and perform these assessments correctly?

Osteomyelitis and Wound Care

@ **Reading Assignment:** Clients with Wounds (Chapter 18)
Management of Clients with Musculoskeletal Disorders
(Chapter 26)

Patient: Harry George, Room 401

Goal: Use the nursing process to competently care for a client with osteomyelitis and a chronic wound.

Objectives:

1. Assess an assigned client for clinical manifestations of osteomyelitis.
2. Describe the causative agent and etiology of osteomyelitis in an assigned client.
3. Safely administer IV antibiotic therapy as prescribed for osteomyelitis.
4. Evaluate diagnostic tests related to osteomyelitis.
5. Develop an appropriate plan of care for a client with a chronic wound.
6. Develop an individualized discharge plan of care for a client with osteomyelitis complicated by other disease processes and homelessness.

Overview:

In this lesson you will learn the essentials of caring for a client with an open wound who is also diagnosed with osteomyelitis. You will explore the client's history, evaluate presenting symptoms and treatment, administer prescribed medications, and develop an individualized discharge teaching plan. Harry George is a 54-year-old male admitted with infection and swelling of his left foot, along with a history of type 2 diabetes, alcohol abuse, and nicotine addiction.

Exercise 1

 Clinical Preparation: Writing Activity

 10 minutes

1. Identify risk factors for osteomyelitis.

2. What is the most common causative organism of osteomyelitis?

3. Identify and describe eight basic concepts of wound assessment and treatment.

Exercise 2

 CD-ROM Activity

 35 minutes

- Sign in to work at Pacific View Regional Hospital for Period of Care 2. (*Note:* If you are already in the virtual hospital from a previous exercise, click on **Leave the Floor** and then **Restart the Program** to get to the sign-in window.)
- From the Patient List, select Harry George (Room 401).
- Click on **Go to Nurses' Station**.
- Click on **Chart** and then on **401**.
- Click on **History and Physical**.

1. The clinical manifestations of osteomyelitis can include both local and systemic symptoms. Common local and systemic signs and symptoms are listed below. Place an X next to any signs or symptoms consistent with Harry George's history and his physical examination findings on admission. Select all that apply.

   _____ a. Acute localized pain

   _____ b. Swelling

   _____ c. Redness

   _____ d. Drainage

   _____ e. Warmth at infection site

   _____ f. Restricted movement

   _____ g. Fever

   _____ h. Nausea

   _____ i. Malaise

   _____ j. Chills

2. Based on what you have read, identify the source (etiology) of Harry George's osteomyelitis. Explain the rationale for your conclusion.

3. What factors in Harry George's history may have contributed to the development of osteomyelitis?

→ • Click on **Physician's Orders**.

4. What diagnositic test(s) did the physician order to evaluate Harry George's osteomyelitis?

→ • Click on **Diagnostic Reports**.

5. Document the findings on the x-ray of Harry George's left foot. Explain the significance of the presence of sequestrum.

→ • Click on **Return to Nurses' Station**.
  • Click on **MAR** and then on tab **401**.

6. Determine what routine medications (excluding the continuous IV and insulin coverage) you will be giving to Harry George during the day shift (0700-1500). Below, list the medications you need to give, the drug classification of each medication, the reason why each is given, and the time each is due. (*Hint:* For help, return to the Nurses' Station and click on the Drug Guide on the counter or click on the **Drug** icon in the lower left corner of your screen.)

Medication	Classification	Reason for Giving	Time Due

7. Which medication was Harry George receiving that was discontinued on Tuesday?

→ • Click on **Return to Nurses' Station**.
  • Click on **Chart** and then on **401**.
  • Click on **Physician's Orders**.

8. What replaced the medication you identified in question 7?

→ • Click on **Physician's Notes**.

9. Why was this change ordered?

 • Click on **Laboratory Reports**.

10. You are aware that the antibiotics have been ordered for Harry George because of his leg infection. You decide to check the WBC results because you are curious (also, you are sure your nursing instructor will ask you about it). Document the WBC results for the times specified below and indicate whether each result is normal, elevated, or decreased.

Tests	Monday 1500	Tuesday 1100	Normal, Elevated, or Decreased?
Total WBC			
Neutrophil segs			
Neutrophil bands			
Lymphocytes			
Monocytes			
Eosinophils			
Basophils			

11. Assessing the data in the above table, explain what the results mean, including the direction of the change in the WBC and the significance of this change.

• Click on **Return to Nurses' Station**.
• Click on **Patient List**.
• Click on **Get Report** for Harry George. Review the report.

12. Is there anything else you wish the nurse would have included in the report regarding osteomyelitis? If so, what?

• Click on **Return to Nurses' Station**.
• Click on **Medication Room**.
• Click on **IV Storage**.
• Click on the **Small Volume** bin and choose the IV antibiotic that is due to be given at 0800.

13. What dilution of this IV antibiotic is available for you to administer?

14. Over what amount of time should you infuse the IV antibiotic? (*Hint:* For help, return to the Nurses' Station and click on the Drug Guide on the counter or click on the **Drug** icon in the lower left corner of your screen.)

15. If you are using an IV pump to deliver this medication piggyback, what rate (mL per hour) will you select to give this infusion?

Exercise 3

 CD-ROM Activity

 40 minutes

• Sign in to work at Pacific View Regional Hospital for Period of Care 2. (*Note:* If you are already in the virtual hospital from a previous exercise, click on **Leave the Floor** and then **Restart the Program** to get to the sign-in window.)
• From the Patient List, select Harry George (Room 401).
• Click on **Go to Nurses' Station** and then on **401** to enter Harry George's room.
• Click on **Take Vital Signs**.

1. Record the vital sign findings below.

BP	SpO$_2$	Temp	HR	RR	Pain

 • Click on **Patient Care** and then **Physical Assesment**.
• Click on **Lower Extremities**.

2. Complete a focused neurovascular and skin assessment of the lower extremities and document your results below.

 • Click on **Patient Care** and then **Nurse-Client Interactions**.
   • Select and view the video titled **1120: Wound Management**. (*Note:* Check the virtual clock to see whether enough time has elapsed. You can use the fast-forward feature to advance the time by 2-minute intervals if the video is not yet available. Then click again on **Patient Care** and **Nurse-Client Interactions** to refresh the screen.)

3. How does the nurse describe the progress of Harry George's wound condition? How does the client respond?

 • Click on **Chart** and then on **401**.
   • Click on **Consultations**.

4. Describe the findings and impressions of the Wound Care Team Consult.

5. What was the recommended plan of care for the wound?

6. Do you have any concerns regarding the above wound care? What different approach might you suggest?

7. What type of nutritional support would be appropriate to enhance wound healing?

- Click on **Return to Room 401**.
- Click on **Medication Room**.
- Click on **MAR** to determine what medications you need to administer to Harry George during this time period (1115-1200).
- Click on **Return to Medication Room**.
- Click on **IV Storage**.
- Click on the **Small Volume** bin and choose the IV antibiotic that is due to be given at 1200.
- Prepare medication by clicking **Put Medication in Tray**.
- Click on **Close Bin**.
- Click on **View Medication Room**.
- Click on the **Drug** icon in the lower left corner of your screen.

8. Look up gentamicin in the Drug Guide. What must you assess before administering this drug? (*Hint:* Look at alert under Administration and Handling.)

→ • Click on **Return to Medication Room**.
  • Click on **Nurses' Station**.
  • Click on **Chart** and then on **401**.
  • Click on **Laboratory Reports**.

9. What are Harry George's most recent peak and trough levels?

10. Based on these results, what should your nursing actions be?

11. For what toxic side effects must you monitor?

12. If Harry George's infection does not respond to the antibiotic therapy or the wound does not heal, what adjunctive treatment might be used? (*Hint:* See page 320 in your textbook.) Explain how these would benefit Harry George.

LESSON 13 ———————————————————

Malnutrition/Obesity

———————————————————————————————

Reading Assignment: Assessment of Nutrition and the Digestive System (Chapter 28)
Management of Clients with Malnutrition (Chapter 29)

Patients: Harry George, Room 401
Jacquline Catanazaro, Room 402
Piya Jordan, Room 403

Goal: Use the nursing process to competently care for clients with nutritional disorders.

Objectives:

1. Identify clients at risk for malnutrition.
2. Perform a nutritional screening assessment on assigned clients.
3. Evaluate laboratory findings in relation to a client's nutritional status.
4. Plan appropriate dietary interventions for a client with malnutrition.
5. Identify a client's risk factors related to obesity.
6. Formulate an appropriate client education plan for an overweight client.

Overview:

In this lesson you will learn the essentials of caring for clients with nutritional disorders. You will explore each client's history, perform a nutritional screening assessment, evaluate findings, and plan appropriate nursing interventions, including the client's educational needs. Harry George is a 54-year-old male with a 4-year history of type 2 diabetes admitted with infection and swelling of his left foot. Piya Jordan is a 68-year-old female admitted with nausea and vomiting for several days following weeks of poor appetite and increasing weakness. Jacquline Catanazaro is a 45-year-old female admitted with an acute exacerbation of asthma.

Exercise 1

 Clinical Preparation: Writing Activity

 10 minutes

1. What are the average caloric and protein needs of a healthy adult?

2. What is the DRI?

3. What do RDA and AI stand for?

4. What is the difference between primary and secondary starvation?

5. Identify and describe the three factors that may lead to obesity.

Exercise 2

 CD-ROM Activity

🕐 40 minutes

- Sign in to work at Pacific View Regional Hospital for Period of Care 1. (*Note:* If you are already in the virtual hospital from a previous exercise, click on **Leave the Floor** and then **Restart the Program** to get to the sign-in window.)
- From the Patient List, select Harry George (Room 401) and Piya Jordan (Room 403).
- Click on **Go to Nurses' Station**.
- Click on **Chart** and then on **401**.
- Click on **History and Physical**.

1. What risk factors for malnutrition are noted in Harry George's H&P?

 • Click on **Return to Nurses' Station**.
- Click on **Chart** and then on **403**.
- Click on **History and Physical**.

2. What risk factors for malnutrition are noted in Piya Jordan's H&P?

 • Click on **Return to Nurses' Station**.
- Click on **401** to enter Harry George's room.
- Click on **Patient Care** and then **Physical Assessment**.

3. Although not every client needs a complete nutritional assessment, it is essential to assess at-risk clients for symptoms of malnutrition. Referring to pages 558-571 of your textbook, assess Harry George for any of the identified findings associated with malnutrition. Obtain subjective information by reading the History and Physical, Nursing Admission, and Laboratory Reports in his chart. Obtain the objective data by completing a physical assessment in his room. Document your findings in column 2 in the table below and on the next page. (*Note:* You will perform a similar assessment on Piya Jordan during Exercise 3 and will record those findings in the third column.)

Screening Assessments	Harry George	Piya Jordan
Health History Biographic and demographic data		
Current Health Chief complaint related to nutrition		
Clinical manifestations		
Past Health History Major illnesses and hospitalizations		
Past surgical procedures		
Allergies		
Medications and dietary supplements		

Screening Assessments	Harry George	Piya Jordan
Dietary habits		
Family health history		
Psychosocial history		

Physical Examination
Height and weight

Body mass index

Mouth

Abdomen

Diagnostic Tests
Serum albumin

CAT scan

4. Evaluate the results of your findings in question 3. Is Harry George malnourished or at risk for malnutrition? Explain how you came to your conclusion.

5. What additional anthropometric measures would be helpful in clarifying Harry George's nutritional status?

6. Is Harry George's protein-energy malnutrition primary or secondary? Explain your answer.

 7. How will Harry George's nutritional status affect the healing of his left foot wound? (*Hint:* See Table 29-1 in your textbook.)

8. What type of diet or dietary supplements would you recommend for Harry George? What nursing interventions might you use to improve his appetite?

Exercise 3

 CD-ROM Activity

 40 minutes

- Sign in to work at Pacific View Regional Hospital for Period of Care 1. (*Note:* If you are already in the virtual hospital from a previous exercise, click on **Leave the Floor** and then **Restart the Program** to get to the sign-in window.)
- From the Patient List, select Harry George (Room 401) and Piya Jordan (Room 403).
- Click on **Go to Nurses' Station** and then on **403** to enter Piya Jordan's room.
- Click on **Patient Care** and then **Physical Assessment**.

 1. Now perform the same nutritional screening assessment on Piya Jordan that you did earlier for Harry George. Referring to pages 558-571 of your textbook, assess Piya Jordan for any of the identified findings associated with malnutrition. Obtain subjective information by reading the History and Physical, Nursing Admission, and Laboratory Reports in her chart. Obtain the objective data by completing a physical assessment in her room. Document your findings in the third column of the table in Exercise 2, question 3.

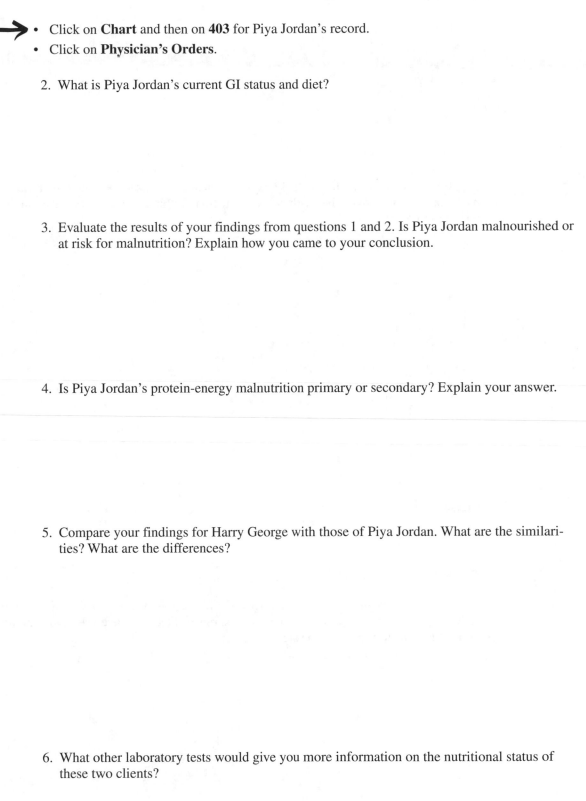

- Click on **Chart** and then on **403** for Piya Jordan's record.
- Click on **Physician's Orders**.

2. What is Piya Jordan's current GI status and diet?

3. Evaluate the results of your findings from questions 1 and 2. Is Piya Jordan malnourished or at risk for malnutrition? Explain how you came to your conclusion.

4. Is Piya Jordan's protein-energy malnutrition primary or secondary? Explain your answer.

5. Compare your findings for Harry George with those of Piya Jordan. What are the similarities? What are the differences?

6. What other laboratory tests would give you more information on the nutritional status of these two clients?

7. Identify two nursing diagnoses related to Piya Jordan's and Harry George's malnourished status.

8. Since Piya Jordan was malnourished on admission and is now NPO, what might the physician order to provide her with needed nutrition? Explain how you would administer this type of nutrition.

Exercise 4

 CD-ROM Activity

 30 minutes

- Sign in to work at Pacific View Regional Hospital for Period of Care 2. (*Note:* If you are already in the virtual hospital from a previous exercise, click on **Leave the Floor** and then **Restart the Program** to get to the sign-in window.)
- From the Patient List, select Jacquline Catanazaro (Room 402).
- Click on **Go to Nurses' Station**.
- Click on **Chart** and then on **402**.
- Click on **Nursing Admission**.

1. Document Jacquline Catanazaro's current height and weight below.

 2. Calculate Jacquline Catanazaro's BMI. (*Hint:* See page 589 in your textbook for the formula.)

3. Is Jacquline Catanazaro's weight normal, overweight, obese, or morbidly obese? (*Hint:* See page 677 in the textbook.)

 • Click on **History and Physical**.

4. What complication of obesity does Jacquline Catanazaro suffer from?

5. What other complications is she at risk for?

6. What are the contributing factors for Jacquline Catanazaro's increased weight?

 • Click on **Return to Nurses' Station**.
   • Click on **MAR** and then on tab **402**.

7. Do any of the medications ordered for Jacquline Catanazaro cause weight gain? If so, explain. (*Hint:* For help, return to the Nurses' Station and click on the Drug Guide on the counter or click on the **Drug** icon in the lower left corner of your screen.)

• Click on **Return to Nurses' Station** and then on **402** to enter the client's room.

- Click on **Patient Care** and then **Nurse-Client Interactions**.
- Select and view the video titled **1140: Compliance—Medications**. (*Note:* Check the virtual clock to see whether enough time has elapsed. You can use the fast-forward feature to advance the time by 2-minute intervals if the video is not yet available. Then click again on **Patient Care** and **Nurse-Client Interactions** to refresh the screen.)

8. What concern does Jacquline Catanazaro voice regarding her medications?

9. Evaluate the nurse's response. Was it appropriate? Accurate?

10. What else could the nurse have suggested to help Jacquline Catanazaro lose weight?

11. If Jacquline Catanazaro had been severely obese (BMI greater than 40), what other treatment options might she have? Briefly explain these options.

LESSON 14

Intestinal Obstruction/ Colorectal Cancer

Reading Assignment: Management of Clients with Intestinal Disorders (Chapter 33)

Patient: Piya Jordan, Room 403

Goal: Use the nursing process to competently care for clients with intestinal disorders.

Objectives:

1. Correlate a client's history and clinical manifestations with a diagnosis of intestinal obstruction.
2. Evaluate laboratory and diagnostic test results of a client admitted with an intestinal disorder.
3. Plan appropriate nursing interventions for a client with a nasogastric tube.
4. Prioritize nursing care for a client with an intestinal obstruction.
5. Provide appropriate psychosocial interventions for a client and family diagnosed with colon cancer.
6. Formulate an appropriate client education plan for a postoperative client with colorectal cancer.

Overview:

In this lesson you will learn the essentials of caring for a client admitted with an intestinal obstruction and diagnosed with colorectal cancer. You will explore the client's history, evaluate presenting symptoms and treatment, plan appropriate nursing interventions, and develop an individualized teaching plan. Piya Jordan is a 68-year-old female admitted with nausea and vomiting for several days following weeks of poor appetite and increasing weakness.

Exercise 1

 Clinical Preparation: Writing Activity

20 minutes

1. Describe the pathophysiology of fluid and electrolyte imbalances associated with an intestinal obstruction.

2. Identify and briefly describe the three categories of etiology related to intestinal obstruction.

3. How does the removal of polyps help to prevent colorectal cancer?

4. Identify the most likely sites of bloodborne metastasis for colorectal cancer.

Exercise 2

 CD-ROM Activity

 40 minutes

- Sign in to work at Pacific View Regional Hospital for Period of Care 1. (*Note:* If you are already in the virtual hospital from a previous exercise, click on **Leave the Floor** and then **Restart the Program** to get to the sign-in window.)
- From the Patient List, select Piya Jordan (Room 403).
- Click on **Go to Nurses' Station**.
- Click on **Chart** and then on **403**.
- Click on **Emergency Department**.

1. What were Piya Jordan's presenting symptoms?

 • Click on **History and Physical**.

2. What history of symptoms is recorded?

 • Click on **Laboratory Reports**.

3. Document Piya Jordan's admission electrolyte results below. Evaluate whether each result is normal, decreased, or increased. Provide rationales for any abnormalities in the last column.

	Monday 2200	Decreased, Normal, or Increased?	Rationale for Abnormality
Sodium			
Potassium			
Chloride			
CO_2			
Creatinine			
BUN			
Amylase			

→ • Click on **Diagnostic Reports**.

4. What was the result of the KUB? What do Piya Jordan's air-fluid levels (gas shadows) indicate?

5. Why do you think a CT scan of the abdomen was ordered? What was the result?

6. What part of the bowel is the terminal ileum?

7. Was Piya Jordan's obstruction mechanical, neurogenic, or vascular? Explain.

8. For what priority problem related to intestinal obstruction should the nurse assess Piya Jordan?

9. If Piya Jordan had sought medical attention before the obstruction occurred, what other diagnostic testing might she have undergone? Explain what the test would show.

➔ • Click on **History and Physical**.

10. Now that you know Piya Jordan has a colonic mass, let's look again at the typical presenting symptoms. Common clinical manifestations of colorectal cancer are listed below. Place an X next to each sign and symptom consistent with Piya Jordan's history and her physical examination findings on admission. Select all that apply.

_____ a. Rectal bleeding

_____ b. Changed bowel habits

_____ c. Blood in stools

_____ d. Anemia

_____ e. Tenesmus

_____ f. Anorexia

_____ g. Nausea and vomiting

_____ h. Fatigue

_____ i. Ribbon-like stools

_____ j. Abdominal pain and cramping

_____ k. Palpable mass

_____ l. Abdominal distention

_____ m. Weight loss

_____ n. Weakness

_____ o. Debility

➔ • Click on **Physician's Orders**.

11. What IV fluid did the ED physician initially order? Why? (*Hint:* Look at the Piya Jordan's vital signs in the Emergency Department Record and relate them to fluid/electrolyte changes noted with intestinal obstruction.)

12. What else did the ED physician order to treat the intestinal obstruction? Explain the purpose of this intervention.

- Click on **Return to Nurses' Station**.
- Click on **403** to enter Piya Jordan's room.
- Click on **Patient Care** and then **Physical Assessment**.

13. Perform a focused abdominal assessment. Document your findings below.

 14. Describe any additional assessments and/or interventions related to the NGT that you might do for Piya Jordan. (*Hint:* See Chapter 31 of your textbook.)

Exercise 3

 CD-ROM Activity

 45 minutes

- Sign in to work at Pacific View Regional Hospital for Period of Care 3. (*Note:* If you are already in the virtual hospital from a previous exercise, click on **Leave the Floor** and then **Restart the Program** to get to the sign-in window.)
- From the Patient List, select Piya Jordan (Room 403).
- Click on **Go to Nurses' Station**.
- Click on **Chart** and then on **403**.
- Click on **History and Physical**.

1. Below is a list of risk factors for colorectal cancer. Place an X next to any that are documented in Piya Jordan's record. Select all that apply.

_____ a. Age

_____ b. History of polyps

_____ c. High-fat, low-residue diet

_____ d. Inflammatory bowel disease

_____ e. Family history

_____ f. History of breast, ovarian, or endometrial cancer

- Click on **Laboratory Reports**.

2. Document Piya Jordan's admission H&H results below. How would you explain the results?

	Monday 2200	Decreased, WNL, or Increased?	Rationale for Abnormality
Hemoglobin			
Hematocrit			

- Click on **Expired MARs**.

3. What was administered preoperatively to clean out Piya Jordan's bowel?

4. If Piya Jordan's surgery had not been an emergency, what type of bowel prep would you have expected to administer? Why is this done?

→ • Click on **Surgical Reports**.

5. Review the operative report. Name and describe the surgical procedure.

6. What is the most likely cell type for Piya Jordan's cancer?

7. How will the physician know what kind of cancer the tumor is?

8. How would you classify Piya Jordan's tumor according to the TNM classification system? Explain.

➤ • Click on **Laboratory Results**.

9. Why did the physician order an amylase, lipase, and LFTs? What do the results demonstrate?

➤ • Click on **Return to Nurses' Station**.
 • Click on **403** to enter Piya Jordan's room.
 • Click on **Patient Care** and then **Nurse-Client Interactions**.
 • Select and view the video titled **1500: Preventing Complications**. (*Note:* Check the virtual clock to see whether enough time has elapsed. You can use the fast-forward feature to advance the time by 2-minute intervals if the video is not yet available. Then click again on **Patient Care** and **Nurse-Client Interactions** to refresh the screen.)

10. What nursing interventions are discussed during this brief video? Why are they appropriate for Piya Jordan?

➤ • Now select and view the video titled **1540: Discharge Planning**. (*Note:* Check the virtual clock to see whether enough time has elapsed. You can use the fast-forward feature to advance the time by 2-minute intervals if the video is not yet available. Then click again on **Patient Care** and **Nurse-Client Interactions** to refresh the screen.)

11. The daughter seems to be overwhelmed by her mother's illness and needs. Describe psychosocial interventions that the nurse might plan to help Piya Jordan and her daughter.

12. What would you teach the daughter regarding health promotion and preventing colon cancer in herself?

13. Identify teaching points that should be discussed with Piya Jordan before her discharge.

LESSON **15** ———————————————————

Diabetes Mellitus

———————————————————

 Reading Assignment: Management of Clients with Diabetes Mellitus (Chapter 45)

Patient: Harry George, Room 401

Goal: Use the nursing process to competently care for clients with diabetes mellitus.

Objectives:

1. Describe the pathophysiology of diabetes mellitus.
2. Compare and contrast the characteristics of type 1 and type 2 diabetes.
3. Identify the relationship between diabetes and other disease processes.
4. Evaluate a client's risk factors for diabetes.
5. Assess a client for short- and long-term complications of diabetes.
6. Develop an appropriate plan of care for a client with type 2 diabetes.

Overview:

In this lesson you will learn the essentials of caring for a client admitted with complications related to diabetes mellitus. You will explore the client's history, evaluate presenting symptoms and treatment, plan appropriate nursing interventions, and develop an individualized teaching plan. Harry George is a 54-year-old male with a 4-year history of type 2 diabetes. He was admitted with infection and swelling of his left foot.

Exercise 1

Clinical Preparation: Writing Activity

20 minutes

1. Describe the pathophysiology of diabetes mellitus and the basis for the resulting abnormalities in carbohydrate, protein, and fat metabolism and utilization.

2. Briefly define and summarize the etiologic differences between type 1 and type 2 diabetes mellitus.

Type 1 diabetes mellitus

Type 2 diabetes mellitus

3. Compare and contrast the distinquishing features of type 1 and type 2 diabetes mellitus (DM) by completing the chart below and on the next page.

Features	Type 1 DM	Type 2 DM
Synonyms		

Features	Type 1 DM	Type 2 DM
Age at onset		
Incidence		
Types of onset		
Endogenous insulin production		
Body weight at onset		
Ketosis		
Manifestations		
Dietary management		
Exercise management		
Exogenous insulin administration		
Oral hypoglycemic agents		

Exercise 2

 CD-ROM Activity

 35 minutes

- Sign in to work at Pacific View Regional Hospital for Period of Care 1. (*Note:* If you are already in the virtual hospital from a previous exercise, click on **Leave the Floor** and then **Restart the Program** to get to the sign-in window.)
- From the Patient List, select Harry George (Room 401).
- Click on **Go to Nurses' Station**.
- Click on **Chart** and then on **401**.
- Click on **History and Physical**.

1. What risk factor(s) for diabetes are noted in Harry George's history?

2. Describe the history of this client's present illness.

3. What is the relationship between the infection in Harry George's foot and his diabetes mellitus? (*Hint:* Read about chronic complications in your textbook.)

→ • Click on **Laboratory Reports**.

4. What was Harry George's admitting blood glucose level?

5. What abnormalities in Harry George's urinalysis results can be attributed to diabetes? Explain the relationship.

→ • Click on **Emergency Department**.

6. What factor in Harry George's recent history most likely contributed to his hyperglycemia? (*Hint:* Read ED physician's notes for 1345.)

7. Listed below are clinical manifestations of diabetes mellitus identified in the textbook. In column 2, indicate (with Yes or No) whether each manifestation is usually present in type 2 diabetes. Then in column 3 indicate (with Yes or No) whether Harry George displays each manifestation based on the nurse's initial assessment.

Clinical Manifestations	Present in Type 2 DM? (Yes or No)	Experienced by Harry George? (Yes or No)
Polyuria		
Polydipsia		
Polyphagia		
Recurrent blurred vision		
Weakness, fatigue, dizziness		
Weight Loss		
Ketonuria		
Pruritus, skin infections		

8. To what extent does Harry George fit the typical picture of a client with type 2 diabetes mellitus?

- Click on **Return to Nurses' Station**.
- Click on **401** to enter Harry George's room.
- Click on **Patient Care** and then **Nurse-Client Interactions**.
- Select and view the video titled **0755: Disease Management**. (*Note:* Check the virtual clock to see whether enough time has elapsed. You can use the fast-forward feature to advance the time by 2-minute intervals if the video is not yet available. Then click again on **Patient Care** and **Nurse-Client Interactions** to refresh the screen.)

9. What does Harry George tell the nurse about his appetite?

→ • Click on **Chart** and then on **401**.
  • Click on **Physician's Orders**.

10. What diet has been ordered for the client?

11. Describe the current recommended nutritional guidelines for the client with diabetes mellitus. (*Hint:* See Table 45-4 in your textbook.)

12. How might the client's alcohol intake affect his blood glucose levels?

13. What complementary therapies might be of benefit to Harry George? Explain. (Hint: See pages 1078 and 1079 in your textbook.)

Exercise 3

  CD-ROM Activity

40 minutes

- Sign in to work at Pacific View Regional Hospital for Period of Care 2. (*Note:* If you are already in the virtual hospital from a previous exercise, click on **Leave the Floor** and then **Restart the Program** to get to the sign-in window.)
- From the Patient List, select Harry George (Room 401).
- Click on **Go to Nurses' Station**.
- Click on **Chart** and then on **401**.
- Click on **Physician's Orders**.

1. What test is ordered that can be used to determine Harry George's control of diabetes mellitus? Describe the purpose of this test. How often should it be done?

2. What was the result of this test for Harry George? Evaluate and explain how well controlled his diabetes is based on these results.

3. What implication does the client's issue of poor glycemic control have for his future?

4. How could Harry George's alcohol intake affect his HgbA$_{1c}$ test result? What implications does this have in managing Harry George's diabetes? How should the nurse intervene?

- Click on **Return to Nurses' Station**.
- Click on **401** to enter Harry George's room.
- Click on **Patient Care** and then **Physical Assessment**.

5. Perform a head-to-toe assessment on Harry George. Document your findings below.

Assessment Area	Assessment Results
Head & Neck	
Chest	
Back & Spine	
Upper Extremities	
Abdomen	
Pelvic	
Lower Extremities	

→ • Click on **EPR** and then on **Login**.
  • Select **401** as the Patient and specify **Neurologic** as the Category.

6. List any abnormal information obtained from the neurologic data recorded on Monday at 1835.

7. Describe the following potential long-term complications for diabetes mellitus.

Coronary artery disease

Cerebrovascular disease

Hypertension

Peripheral vascular disease

Retinopathy

Nephropathy

Neuropathy

8. Does Harry George exhibit any signs that would alert you to the possibility of any of the long-term complications noted in question 7? If so, explain. (*Hint:* Review your responses to questions 5 and 6 of this exercise and also consider your response to question 5 in Exercise 2.)

9. What client teaching would you plan to offer Harry George to prevent injury secondary to reduced sensation in his left foot?

10. Using correct NANDA format, state three nursing diagnoses related to Harry George's diabetes.

LESSON **16** ————————————————————

Hypertension

———————————————————————————

Reading Assignment: Management of Clients with Hypertensive Disorders
(Chapter 52)

Patients: Harry George, Room 401
Patricia Newman, Room 406

Goal: Use the nursing process to competently care for clients with hypertension.

Objectives:

1. Describe the four classifications of blood pressure.
2. Identify the presence of risk factors for hypertension in assigned clients.
3. Discuss pharmacologic therapies available to treat hypertension.
4. Develop an extensive educational plan for clients with hypertension.
5. Discuss appropriate care for a client in an acute hypertension crisis.

Overview:

In this lesson you will learn the essentials of caring for a client with hypertension. You will explore the client's history, evaluate presenting symptoms and treatment, identify blood pressure classification, provide appropriate nursing interventions, and plan an appropriate client education plan related to the hypertension. Patricia Newman is a 61-year-old female admitted with pneumonia and a history of emphysema. Harry George is a 54-year-old male admitted with infection and swelling of the left foot.

Exercise 1

Clinical Preparation: Writing Activity

20 minutes

1. Identify and describe the four classifications of blood pressure.

2. Describe how the the following control systems work to maintain blood pressure.

   a. Arterial baroreceptor and chemoreceptors system

   b. Regulation of body fluid volume

   c. Renin-angiotensin system

d. Vascular autoregulation

3. Define the following terms.

a. Primary hypertension

b. Secondary hypertension

c. Isolated systolic hypertension (ISH)

e. Resistant hypertension

4. Identify four nonmodifiable risk factors for hypertension.

5. Identify six modifiable risk factors for hypertension.

Exercise 2

 CD-ROM Activity

 45 minutes

- Sign in to work at Pacific View Regional Hospital for Period of Care 1. (*Note:* If you are already in the virtual hospital from a previous exercise, click on **Leave the Floor** and then **Restart the Program** to get to the sign-in window.)
- From the Patient List, select Patricia Newman (Room 406).
- Click on **Go to Nurses' Station**.
- Click on **Chart** and then on **406**.
- Click on **History and Physical**.

1. How long ago was Patricia Newman diagnosed with hypertension?

 • Click on **Nursing Admission**.

2. What risk factors for hypertension does Patricia Newman have?

 • Click on **Physician's Orders**.

3. In the table below, identify the two medications ordered to treat Patricia Newman's hypertension. For each one, identify the drug classification and mechanism of action. You will complete the table in questions 4 and 5. (*Hint:* You may consult the Drug Guide in the Nurses' Station.)

Medication	Drug Classification	Mechanism of Action	Nursing Assessments	Common Side Effects

 • Click on **Return to Nurses' Station**.
• Click on the **Drug** icon in the lower left corner of the screen.

4. What nursing assessments are important to complete before administering the medications you identified in question 3? Record your answer in the fourth column of the table in quesion 3.

5. For what side effects will the nurse need to monitor the client? Record your answer in the last column of the table in question 3.

→ • Click on **Return to Nurses' Station**; then select **EPR** and click on **Login**.
 • Select **406** from the Patient menu and specify **Vital Signs** as the Category.

6. What are Patricia Newman's documented blood pressure measurements since admission?

7. Is her prescribed antihypertensive medication currently effective?

8. In what classification would you put Patricia Newman's blood pressure based on her most current readings? Explain.

→ • Click on **Exit EPR**.
 • Click on **406** to go to Patricia Newman's room.
 • Click on **Patient Care** and then **Nurse-Client Interactions**.
 • Select and view the video titled **0740: Evaluation—Response to Care**. (*Note:* Check the virtual clock to see whether enough time has elapsed. You can use the fast-forward feature to advance the time by 2-minute intervals if the video is not yet available. Then click again on **Patient Care** and **Nurse-Client Interactions** to refresh the screen.)

9. What might be contributing to Patricia Newman's currently elevated blood pressure?

→ • Click on **Chart** and then on **406**.
 • Click on **History and Physical**.

10. What indicates that Patricia Newman is in need of further teaching regarding hypertension?

→ • Click on **Patient Education**.

11. What additional educational goals would be appropriate for Patricia Newman?

12. Develop a comprehensive individualized teaching plan for Patricia Newman regarding nonpharmacologic measures to treat hypertension.

→ • Click on **Nursing Admission**.

13. Was Patricia Newman following any of the interventions you identified in question 12 to reduce her blood pressure at home? Explain.

→ • Click on **Physician's Orders**.

14. Identify any of the interventions addressed in question 12 that were ordered for Patricia Newman during this hospital stay.

15. As the nurse caring for Patricia Newman, what do you think would be your professional responsibility related to your findings for questions 13 and 14?

Exercise 3

 CD-ROM Activity

 40 minutes

• Sign in to work at Pacific View Regional Hospital for Period of Care 1. (*Note:* If you are already in the virtual hospital from a previous exercise, click on **Leave the Floor** and then **Restart the Program** to get to the sign-in window.)
• From the Patient List, select Harry George (Room 401).
• Click on **Go to Nurses' Station**.

• Click on **EPR** and then on **Login**.
   • Select **401** as the Patient and **Vital Signs** as the Category.

1. Document Harry George's blood pressures (BP) for the times listed below.

	Tues 0305	Tues 0705	Tues 1105	Tues 1505	Tues 1905	Tues 2305	Wed 0305	Wed 0705
BP								

➤ • Click on **Exit EPR**.
   • Click on **Chart** and then on **401**.
   • Click on **History and Physical**.

2. Does Harry George have a history of hypertension?

3. Does he have any risk factors for hypertension? If yes, please identify.

4. Based on the BP recordings you documented in question 1, in what classification would you put Harry George's blood pressure?

5. For what potential target organ damage should you assess related to untreated hypertension?

• Click on **Return to Nurses' Station**.
 • Click on **401**.
 • Click on **Patient Care** and then **Physical Assessment**.
 • Select the various assessment areas (yellow buttons) and system subcategories (green buttons) as needed to answer question 6.

6. Listed below are physical assessment findings indicative of target organ damage from hypertension. Place an X next to any that you noted during your physical assessment of Harry George. Select all that apply.

_____ a. Distended neck veins

_____ b. Enlarged thyroid

_____ c. Dysrhythmias

_____ d. Murmurs

_____ e. Abdominal bruit

_____ f. Edema

_____ g. Carotid bruits

_____ h. Increased heart rate

_____ i. Precordial impulses

_____ j. S_3 and S_4 heart sounds

_____ k. Diminished or absent peripheral pulses

_____ l. Bilateral inequality of pulses

7. What target organ disease is consistent with the above findings?

8. Several diagnostic tests were ordered by the physician (listed below and on the next page). Although these tests may have been ordered for various purposes, they may specifically help to identify target organ disease. In the middle column, indicate how each test might be helpful. (*Note:* You will complete this table in questions 9 and 10.)

Diagnostic Test	How Test Might Help Identify Target Organ Disease	Results
Chest x-ray		

Diagnostic Test	How Test Might Help Identify Target Organ Disease	Results
BUN		
Creatinine		
Urinalysis		

➡ • Click on **Chart** and then **401**.
  • Click on **Diagnostic Reports**.

9. Record the results of Harry George's chest x-ray in the third column of the table in question 8 and indicate whether or not the results suggest the presence of target organ disease.

➡ • Click on **Laboratory Reports**.

10. Find and record the lab results for BUN, creatinine, and urinalysis in the table in question 8. Indicate what these results mean related to target organ disease.

11. What would be the first step in treating Harry George's hypertension?

12. If the above interventions failed to lower Harry George's blood pressure to normal limits, what classification of drugs might the health care provider prescribe?

13. If Harry George continues to have inadequate blood pressure control, what other drug classifications might the health care provider add to the client's therapeutic regimen?

14. If Harry George's blood pressure would suddenly increase to 260/160 mm Hg, what symptoms of hypertensive crisis would you assess him for?

Atrial Fibrillation

Reading Assignment: Assessment of the Cardiac System (Chapter 54)
Management of Clients with Functional Cardiac Disorders
(Chapter 56)
Management of Clients with Dysrhythmias (Chapter 57)

Patient: Piya Jordan, Room 403

Goal: Use the nursing process to competently care for clients with dysrhythmias.

Objectives:

1. Describe rhythm strip characteristics of atrial fibrillation.
2. Identify potential etiologic causes of atrial fibrillation for an assigned client.
3. Assess a client for clinical manifestations of atrial fibrillation.
4. Develop a plan of care to monitor a client for potential complications of atrial fibrillation.
5. Perform appropriate assessments prior to administering pharmacologic therapy for atrial fibrillation.
6. Accurately administer IV digoxin.
7. Discuss the use of anticoagulation therapy for a client with atrial fibrillation.
8. Develop appropriate educational outcomes for a client with a history of atrial fibrillation.

Overview:

In this lesson you will learn the essentials of caring for a client with a cardiac dysrhythmia. You will explore the client's history, evaluate presenting symptoms and treatment, provide appropriate nursing interventions, and plan an appropriate client educational outcome related to the dysrhythmia. Piya Jordan is a 68-year-old female admitted with nausea, vomiting, and abdominal pain.

Exercise 1

Clinical Preparation: Writing Activity

20 minutes

1. Briefly describe the three pathophysiologic mechanisms that can cause dysrhythmias.

2. Describe the concept of atrial kick. Why is this important?

3. Identify the cardiac event represented by each of the following waves.

   a. P wave

   b. QRS wave

   c. T wave

4. Describe the seven steps of ECG analysis, as identified in your textbook.

   a.

   b.

   c.

d.

e.

f.

g.

Exercise 2

 CD-ROM Activity

 35 minutes

- Sign in to work at Pacific View Regional Hospital for Period of Care 1. (*Note:* If you are already in the virtual hospital from a previous exercise, click on **Leave the Floor** and then **Restart the Program** to get to the sign-in window.)
- From the Patient List, select Piya Jordan (Room 403).
- Click on **Go to Nurses' Station**.
- Click on **403** to enter Piya Jordan's room.

1. What information regarding Piya Jordan's cardiovascular status is obtained on initial observation of the client?

2. What is atrial fibrillation?

3. Describe the rhythm strip you would expect to see on Piya Jordan's monitor.

4. How does this differ from normal sinus rhythm?

5. What effect does this rhythm have on cardiac output? Explain.

6. For what clinical manifestations related to atrial fibrillation should you monitor Piya Jordan?

→ • Click on **Patient Care** and then on **Physical Assessment**. Perform a general assessment of Piya Jordan.

7. Are any of the symptoms you listed in question 6 present in Piya Jordan? If not, how would you explain that?

8. If Piya Jordan's heart rate increases, how might the atrial fibrillation affect her blood pressure? Describe the underlying physiology. (*Hint:* Think about the atrial kick.)

→ • Click on **Chart** and then on **403**.
  • Click on **Diagnostic Reports**.

9. Did Piya Jordan have a 12-lead ECG done? If yes, what was the rhythm? If not, do you think it should have been done? Why or why not?

10. For what potential complications should you monitor Piya Jordan?

Exercise 3

 CD-ROM Activity

 45 minutes

- Sign in to work at Pacific View Regional Hospital for Period of Care 1. (*Note:* If you are already in the virtual hospital from a previous exercise, click on **Leave the Floor** and then **Restart the Program** to get to the sign-in window.)
- From the Patient List, select Piya Jordan (Room 403).
- Click on **Go to Nurses' Station**.
- Click on **MAR** and then on tab **403** for Piya Jordan's record.

1. What medication is prescribed to treat Piya Jordan's atrial fibrillation? Describe the pharmacodynamics of this medication as related to atrial fibrillation. (*Hint:* For help, return to the Nurses' Station and click on the Drug Guide on the counter or on the **Drug** icon in the lower left corner of your screen.)

2. Why did the physician order a digoxin level when the client first presented to the ED? (*Hint:* Review her presenting symptoms, as well as the Drug Guide.)

 • Click on **Return to Nurses' Station**.
- Click on **Chart** and then on **403**.
- Click on **Laboratory Reports**.

3. What was Piya Jordan's digoxin level in the ED? Is this therapeutic or toxic?

4. For what other symptoms would you monitor Piya Jordan in relation to digoxin toxicity?

5. What was the client's potassium level on admission to the ED?

6. How does this relate to possible digoxin toxicity?

→ • Click on **History and Physical**.

7. What other medication was Piya Jordan prescribed related to atrial fibrillation before this admission? Provide a rationale for this medication. (*Hint:* Think of potential serious complications of atrial fibrillation.)

→ • Click on **Physician's Orders**.

8. What two items did the physician prescribe preoperatively to reverse Piya Jordan's anti-coagulation? How would you know this was effective? Please explain.

9. What was ordered postoperatively to prevent clot formation?

→ • Click on **Nursing Admission**.

10. What knowledge (or lack of knowledge) does Piya Jordan verbalize regarding her history of atrial fibrillation? (*Hint:* Check the Health Promotion section.)

→ • Click on **Patient Education** and review the expected outcomes.

11. What might you add to these outcomes relative to your answer to question 10?

12. What other pharmaceutical options are available to treat Piya Jordan's atrial fibrillation?

13. Explain how electrical cardioversion might benefit Piya Jordan.

14. What preparation would Piya Jordan need if she were to undergo electrical cardioversion?

15. What interventional therapy may be used for clients with recurrent or sustained atrial fibrillation?

Now it's time to prepare and administer Piya Jordan's ordered medications.

Medication Preparation

- Click on **Return to Nurses' Station**.
- Click on **Medication Room**.
- Click on **MAR** to determine medications that Piya Jordan is ordered to receive at 0800. (*Note:* You may click on **Review MAR** at any time to verify correct medication order. Remember to look at the patient name on the MAR to make sure you have the correct patient's record—you must click on the correct room number within the MAR. Click on **Return to Medication Room** after reviewing the correct MAR.)
- Based on your care for Piya Jordan, access the various storage areas of the Medication Room to obtain the necessary medications you need to administer.
- For each area you access, first select the medication you would like to administer, then click **Put Medication on Tray**. When finished with a storage area, click on **Close Drawer**.
- Click **View Medication Room**.
- Click on **Preparation** and choose the correct medication to administer. Click **Prepare**.
- Click **Next** and choose the correct patient to administer this medication to. Click **Finish**.
- Repeat the above two steps until all medications that you want to administer are prepared.
- You can click **Review Your Medications** and then **Return to Medication Room** when you are ready. Once you are back in the Medication Room, you may go directly to Piya Jordan's room by clicking on **403** at the bottom of the screen.

Medication Administration

- Administer the medication, utilizing the five rights of medication administration. After you have collected the appropriate assessment data and are ready for administration, click **Patient Care** and then **Medication Administration**. Verify that the correct patient and medication(s) appear in the left-hand window. Then click the down arrow next to Select. From the drop-down menu, select **Administer** and complete the Administration Wizard by providing any information requested. When the Wizard stops asking for information, click **Administer to Patient**. Specify **Yes** when asked whether this administration should be recorded in the MAR. Finally, click **Finish**.

16. Over how many minutes would you administer the IV digoxin?

17. What should you have assessed before administering digoxin to Piya Jordan today?

Now let's see how you did!

 • Click on **Leave the Floor** at the bottom of your screen. From the Floor Menu, select **Look at Your Preceptor's Evaluation**. Then click on **Medication Scorecard**.

18. Note below whether or not you correctly administered the appropriate medications. If not, why do you think you were incorrect? According to Table C in this scorecard, what resources should be used and what assessments should be completed before administering the medications? Did you use these resources and perform these assessments correctly?

LESSON **18** ──────────────────────

Asthma

───────────────────────────────────────

Reading Assignment: Management of Clients with Lower Airway and Pulmonary Vessel Disorders (Chapter 61)

Patient: Jacquline Catanazaro, Room 402

Goal: Use the nursing process to competently care for clients with asthma.

Objectives:

1. Identify clinical manifestations of an acute asthmatic exacerbation.
2. Evaluate diagnostic tests as they relate to a client's oxygenation status.
3. Describe medications used to treat asthma, including mechanism of action and therapeutic effects.
4. Prioritize nursing care for a client with an acute exacerbation of asthma.
5. Formulate an appropriate client education plan regarding home asthma management for a client with identified barriers to learning.

Overview:

In this lesson you will learn the essentials of caring for a client diagnosed with asthma. You will explore the client's history, evaluate presenting symptoms and treatment upon admission, and follow the client's progress throughout the hospital stay. Jacquline Catanazaro is a 45-year-old female admitted with increasing respiratory distress. Begin this lesson by reviewing the general concepts of asthma as presented in your textbook.

Exercise 1

 Clinical Preparation: Writing Activity

30 minutes

1. What is another name for asthma?

2. Briefly describe the pathophysiology of asthma.

3. Compare and contrast the four classifications and steps of asthma management by completing the table below.

Steps of Asthma	Symptoms	Nighttime Symptoms	Preferred Treatment Recommendations
Step 4 Severe persistent			
Step 3 Moderate persistent			
Step 2 Mild persistent			
Step 1 Mild intermittent			

4. Define the following pulmonary function test measurements. (*Hint:* See "Pulmonary Function Test [PFT] Components" on the Evolve site for Chapter 59.)

   a. Forced vital capacity (FVC)

   b. Forced expiratory volume in the first second (FEV_1)

   c. Peak expiratory flow rate (PEFR)

5. What is a normal PEFR reading?

Exercise 2

 CD-ROM Activity

 40 minutes

- Sign in to work at Pacific View Regional Hospital for Period of Care 1. (*Note:* If you are already in the virtual hospital from a previous exercise, click on **Leave the Floor** and then **Restart the Program** to get to the sign-in window.)
- From the Patient List, select Jacquline Catanazaro (Room 402).
- Click on **Go to Nurses' Station**.
- Click on **Chart** and then on **402**.
- Click on **History and Physical**.

1. What medical problems does Jacquline Catanazaro have?

2. What pathologic triggers can lead to an exacerbation of asthma?

3. Does Jacquline Catanazaro's history identify any of these triggers?

4. What other factor(s) might be contributing to Jacquline Catanazaro's asthma exacerbations?

5. Based on Jacquline Catanazaro's history and home medication regimen, what step of asthma management do you think she is normally at (excluding this admission for an exacerbation)? Explain.

➡ • Click on **Emergency Department**.

6. What were Jacquline Catanazaro's presenting symptoms?

7. What diagnostic testing was ordered? Document and interpret the abnormal results below. (*Hint:* Review Laboratory Reports and Diagnostic Reports to obtain these results.)

8. Read the ED physician's progress notes for 1400. What are the results of the client's PEFR? How would you interpret these in light of her present condition?

→ • Click on **Physician's Orders**.

9. What medical treatment is ordered in the ED? (*Hint:* See orders for Monday at 1005.)

10. How would you evaluate the client's response to medical treatment?

11. What medications were ordered on Monday at 1600? What is the mechanism of action for each of these drugs? (*Hint:* Return to the Nurses' Station and click on the Drug Guide on the counter or on the **Drug** icon in the lower left corner of your screen.)

12. Do these medications need to be administered in any specific order? Explain.

13. What new medications are ordered on Tuesday at 0800? Provide a rationale for these orders. Why is the prednisone ordered to be decreased by 5 mg every day?

Exercise 3

 CD-ROM Activity

 30 minutes

- Sign in to work at Pacific View Regional Hospital for Period of Care 1. (*Note:* If you are already in the virtual hospital from a previous exercise, click on **Leave the Floor** and then **Restart the Program** to get to the sign-in window.)
- From the Patient List, select Jacquline Catanazaro (Room 402).
- Click on **Go to Nurses' Station**.
- Click on **402**.
- Read the **Initial Observations**.

1. Describe what you learn from the Initial Observations when you enter Jacquline Catanazaro's room.

 • Click on **Take Vital Signs**.

2. Record Jacquline Catanazaro's vital signs below.

3. Are there any Clinical Alerts for Jacquline Catanazaro? If so, describe below.

4. How would you prioritize your care for the client at this point?

→ • Click on **Patient Care** and then **Physical Assessment**.

5. Perform a focused assessment on three priority areas based on Jacquline Catanazaro's present status. Document your findings below.

Focused Areas of Assessment	Jacquline Catanazaro's Assessment Findings
a.	
b.	
c.	

→ • Click on **Chart** and then on **402**.
• Click on **Physician's Orders**.

6. What new orders did the physician write on Monday at 0730?

→ • Click on **Return to Room 402**.
• Click on **Patient Care** and then **Nurse-Client Interactions**.
• Select and view the video titled **0730: Intervention—Airway**. (*Note:* Check the virtual clock to see whether enough time has elapsed. You can use the fast-forward feature to advance the time by 2-minute intervals if the video is not yet available. Then click again on **Patient Care** and **Nurse-Client Interactions** to refresh the screen.)

7. How does the nurse in this video prioritize her actions? Give a rationale for these actions.

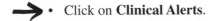 • Click on **Clinical Alerts**.

8. Look at the 0800 Clinical Alert. Interpret this alert below.

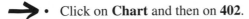 • Click on **Chart** and then on **402**.
• Click on **Physician's Notes**.

9. Read the notes for Wednesday at 0800. How does the physician evaluate the client's condition at this point?

➤ • Click on **Physician's Orders**.

10. Below, record the orders for 0800 on Wednesday. Provide a rationale or expected therapeutic response for each order.

New Orders	Rationale/Expected Therapeutic Response

Exercise 4

 CD-ROM Activity

 45 minutes

- Sign in to work at Pacific View Regional Hospital for Period of Care 2. (*Note:* If you are already in the virtual hospital from a previous exercise, click on **Leave the Floor** and then **Restart the Program** to get to the sign-in window.)
- From the Patient List, select Jacquline Catanazaro (Room 402).
- Click on **Get Report**.

1. Briefly summarize the activity for Jacquline Catanazaro over the last 4 hours.

 • Click on **Go to Nurses' Station**.
  - Click on **402** to go to the patient's room.

2. What is your initial observation of Jacquline Catanazaro for this time period?

3. Are there any clinical alerts?

→ • Click on **Take Vital Signs**.

4. Record the client's vital signs below. How do these results compare with those you obtained during Period of Care 1? (*Hint:* See Exercise 3, question 2 of this lesson.)

→ • Click on **Patient Care** and then **Physical Assessment**.

5. Perform a focused assessment on Jacquline Catanazaro and record your findings in the middle column below and on the next page. In the last column, compare these current findings with those you obtained during Period of Care 1. Interpret your results. (*Hint:* See Exercise 3, question 5.)

Focused Areas of Assessment	Current Findings	Comparison with 0800 Findings—Interpretation of Results
Respiratory		
Cardiovascular		

Focused Areas of Assessment	Current Findings	Comparison with 0800 Findings— Interpretation of Results
Mental Status		

 • Click on **Patient Care** and then **Nurse-Client Interactions**.

• Select and view the video titled **1115: Assessment—Readiness to Learn**. (*Note:* Check the virtual clock to see whether enough time has elapsed. You can use the fast-forward feature to advance the time by 2-minute intervals if the video is not yet available. Then click again on **Patient Care** and **Nurse-Client Interactions** to refresh the screen.)

6. Describe the nurse's actions in the video. Are they appropriate? Explain.

7. What barriers to learning might be present for Jacquline Catanazaro?

 • Click on **Leave the Floor**.

• Click on **Restart the Program**.

• Sign in for Period of Care 3.

• From the Patient List, select Jacquline Catanazaro (Room 402).

• Click on **Go to Nurses' Station** and then on **402** to enter the patient's room.

• Click on **Patient Care** and then **Nurse-Client Interactions**.

• Select and view the video titled **1500: Intervention—Patient Teaching**. (*Note:* Check the virtual clock to see whether enough time has elapsed. You can use the fast-forward feature to advance the time by 2-minute intervals if the video is not yet available. Then click again on **Patient Care** and **Nurse-Client Interactions** to refresh the screen.)

8. In the video, what equipment is the nurse teaching the client about?

9. Describe the proper use of the peak flow meter for this client.

10. What should Jacquline Catanazaro be taught regarding the results of her peak flow measurements?

11. Describe the directions you would give Jacquline Catanazaro for properly using a metered-dose inhaler (MDI).

12. What other asthma management needs would you teach the client?

➡ • Click on **Chart** and then on **402**.
  • Click on **Patient Education**.

13. What are the educational goals for Jacquline Catanazaro?

14. Describe the differences in outcomes met for the client and her sister.

15. The client is scheduled for discharge tomorrow. Do you have any concerns? What would be your most appropriate action?

LESSON 19

DVT/Pulmonary Embolism

 Reading Assignment: Management of Clients with Vascular Disorders (Chapter 53)
Management of Clients with Lower Airway and
Pulmonary Vessel Disorders (Chapter 61)

Patient: Clarence Hughes, Room 404

Goal: Use the nursing process to competently care for clients with a critically altered oxygenation state.

Objectives:

1. Identify clinical manifestations of pulmonary embolism.
2. Prioritize nursing care for a client with acute onset of respiratory distress and chest pain.
3. Describe diagnostic testing relative to the diagnosis of pulmonary embolism.
4. Describe pharmacologic therapy for a client with pulmonary embolism.
5. Accurately calculate correct dosage of heparin for a client by using a sliding scale.
6. Identify disease management issues regarding the care of a client with a pulmonary embolism.

Overview:

In this lesson you will learn the essentials of caring for a client diagnosed with an acute pulmonary embolism as a sequela of deep vein thrombosis. You will explore the client's history, evaluate presenting symptoms and treatment, provide appropriate nursing interventions, and assess the client's progress throughout the clinical day. Clarence Hughes is a 73-year-old male admitted for an elective left knee arthroplasty.

Exercise 1

 Clinical Preparation: Writing Activity

10 minutes

1. What is Virchow's triad?

2. Describe nursing interventions used to prevent DVT in at-risk clients.

Exercise 2

 CD-ROM Activity

 30 minutes

- Sign in to work at Pacific View Regional Hospital for Period of Care 2. (*Note:* If you are already in the virtual hospital from a previous exercise, click on **Leave the Floor** and then **Restart the Program** to get to the sign-in window.)
- From the Patient List, select Clarence Hughes (Room 404).
- Click on **Get Report**.

1. Before entering Clarence Hughes' room, summarize what you would expect to find based on the report you received.

- Click on **Go to Nurses' Station**.
- Click on **404** to go to Clarence Hughes' room.

2. What is your initial observation as you enter the client's room?

3. What should your priority actions be at this point?

 • Click on **Patient Care** and then **Nurse-Client Interactions**.
  • Select and view the video titled **1115: Interventions—Airway**. (*Note:* Check the virtual clock to see whether enough time has elapsed. You can use the fast-forward feature to advance the time by 2-minute intervals if the video is not yet available. Then click again on **Patient Care** and **Nurse-Client Interactions** to refresh the screen.)

4. Describe the nurse's actions in this video. Should the nurse have left the client to go get oxygen? Explain your answer. If not, what else could she have done?

5. What clinical manifestations of pulmonary embolus is Clarence Hughes displaying?

6. Suspecting a pulmonary embolus, what other clinical manifestations would you assess Clarence Hughes for?

• Click on **Chart** and then on **404**.
 • Click on **History and Physical**.

7. Based on the client's history and current reason for hospitalization, what risk factors for DVT and resultant pulmonary embolus does Clarence Hughes have?

 • Click on **Physician's Orders**.

8. Look at the orders dated Wednesday at 1120. Document these orders below and provide a rationale for each.

Physician Order	Rationale

• Click on **Return to Room 404**.
  • Click on **Patient Care** and then on **Nurse-Client Interactions**.
  • Select and view the video titled **1135: Change in Patient Condition**. (*Note:* Check the virtual clock to see whether enough time has elapsed. You can use the fast-forward feature to advance the time by 2-minute intervals if the video is not yet available. Then click again on **Patient Care** and **Nurse-Client Interactions** to refresh the screen.)

9. As the nurse in the video explains care to the family, she states that a transporter will be coming to take Clarence Hughes for a ventilation-perfusion scan. Would you send this client down to radiology with just the transporter? Why or why not?

Exercise 3

 CD-ROM Activity

 30 minutes

  • Sign in to work at Pacific View Regional Hospital for Period of Care 3. (*Note:* If you are already in the virtual hospital from a previous exercise, click on **Leave the Floor** and then **Restart the Program** to get to the sign-in window.)
  • From the Patient List, select Clarence Hughes (Room 404).
  • Click on **Go to Nurses' Station**.
  • Click on **Chart** and then on **404**.
  • Click on **Laboratory Reports** and **Diagnostic Reports**.

1. In the table below, list the tests and results you found in Clarence Hughes' chart.

Diagnostic Test	Result

2. Based on the results you documented in question 1, what would you conclude to be the cause of Clarence Hughes' acute respiratory distress?

3. Name four other diagnostic tests the physician could have ordered related to Clarence Hughes' embolism.

➤ • Click on **Physician's Orders**.

4. What orders were written to treat Clarence Hughes' pulmonary embolus?

5. What lab test will be used to titrate the heparin infusion?

6. What is the desired therapeutic level for this lab test? (*Hint:* You may consult the Drug Guide in the Nurses' Station.)

➤ • Click on **Return to Nurses' Station**.
   • Click on **MAR** and then on **404**.

7. How many units of heparin would you administer for the bolus dose?

8. If you were the nurse starting the heparin infusion, at what rate would you set the IV pump to infuse this medication?

 • Click on **Return to Nurses' Station**.
 • Click on **Chart** and then on **404**.
 • Click on **Laboratory Reports**.

9. What were the results of the aPTT and INR at 1300 today? Why were these tests ordered prior to starting the heparin?

 • Click on **Return to Nurses' Station**.
 • Click on **404** to enter Clarence Hughes' room.
 • Click on **Patient Care** and then on **Patient-Client Interactions**.
 • Select and view the video titled **1510: Disease Management**. (*Note:* Check the virtual clock to see whether enough time has elapsed. You can use the fast-forward feature to advance the time by 2-minute intervals if the video is not yet available. Then click again on **Patient Care** and **Nurse-Client Interactions** to refresh the screen.)

10. When the son asks the nurse whether the pulmonary embolism would delay his father's discharge, the nurse states that the heparin takes 2 days to stabilize. Does this mean that the client will be discharged on heparin? If not, what medication will be used to minimize clot formation? Explain why the client will not be started on this medication rather than heparin.

11. What lab test(s) will be used to monitor the therapeutic effect of Coumadin? What is the therapeutic range for these tests?

12. For what possible complications would you monitor Clarence Hughes related to the pulmonary embolism?

20

Emphysema and Pneumonia

Reading Assignment: Management of Clients with Lower Airway and
Pulmonary Vessel Disorders (Chapter 61)
Management of Clients with Parenchymal and
Pleural Disorders (Chapter 62)

Patient: Patricia Newman, Room 406

Goal: Use the nursing process to competently care for clients with altered oxygenation states.

Objectives:

1. Relate physical assessment findings with pathophysiologic changes of the lower respiratory
   tract.
2. Prioritize nursing care for a client with altered oxygenation.
3. Evaluate laboratory results relative to the diagnosis of pneumonia and emphysema.
4. Describe pharmacologic interventions related to altered oxygenation states.
5. Identify appropriate nursing interventions for a client admitted with pneumonia and
   emphysema.
6. Identify appropriate discharge teaching needs for a client with altered oxygenation.

Overview:

In this lesson you will learn the essentials of caring for a client diagnosed with pneumonia and
emphysema. You will explore the client's history, evaluate presenting symptoms and treatment
upon admission, and assess the client's progress throughout the hospital stay. Patricia Newman
is a 61-year-old female admitted with pneumonia and a history of emphysema. Begin this lesson
by first reviewing the general concepts of altered oxygenation states as presented in your textbook.

Exercise 1

Clinical Preparation: Writing Activity

20 minutes

1. What category of lung diseases does emphysema belong to?

2. Briefly describe the pathophysiology of emphysema.

3. Briefly describe the pathophysiology of pneumonia.

4. What are the major risk factors for pneumonia?

Exercise 2

 CD-ROM Activity

 45 minutes

- Sign in to work at Pacific View Regional Hospital for Period of Care 1. (*Note:* If you are already in the virtual hospital from a previous exercise, click on **Leave the Floor** and then **Restart the Program** to get to the sign-in window.)
- From the Patient List, select Patricia Newman (Room 406).
- Click on **Get Report**.

1. What questions would you ask the outgoing nurses to obtain needed information not identified in report?

2. Below, relate the clinical manifestations identified in the change-of-shift report to the client's diagnosis of pneumonia.

Clinical Manifestations	Pathophysiologic Basis
Labored respirations	
Use of accessory muscles	
Productive cough with yellow sputum	
Coarse breath sounds	
Lung infiltrates	
Disturbed sleep patterns	
Tachycardia	
Fever	

→ • Click on **Go to Nurses' Station**.
  • Click on **Chart** and then on **406**.
  • Click on **History and Physical**.

3. What risk factors for pneumonia does Patricia Newman have?

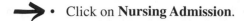• Click on **Nursing Admission**.

4. What other risk factor for pneumonia is documented on the Nursing Admission form? (*Hint:* Look for something that might have prevented the pneumonia.)

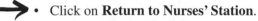• Click on **Return to Nurses' Station**.
• Click on **406** to enter Patricia Newman's room.
• Click on **Initial Observations**.

5. What would be your priority nursing assessment/intervention(s) based on the Initial Observations?

• Click on **Patient Care** and then **Physical Assessment**.

6. Perform a focused clinical assessment based on Patricia Newman's admitting diagnosis and record your findings below. How has Patricia Newman's condition changed since report?

Focused Assessment Area	Assessment Findings	Change in Assessment

 • Click on **Patient Care** and then **Nurse-Client Interactions**.

• Select and view the video titled **0730: Prioritizing Interventions**. (*Note:* Check the virtual clock to see whether enough time has elapsed. You can use the fast-forward feature to advance the time by 2-minute intervals if the video is not yet available. Then click again on **Patient Care** and **Nurse-Client Interactions** to refresh the screen.)

7. Evaluate the nurse's actions based on the client's current status. How does this nurse's action differ from your plan of care as answered in question 5?

8. Identify appropriate nursing interventions to maintain effective airway clearance and breathing pattern for Patricia Newman.

9. What nursing interventions might alleviate Patricia Newman's anxiety and improve her activity tolerance?

→ • Click on **Chart** and then on **406**.
 • Click on **Laboratory Reports**.

10. Identify any abnormal lab results and describe how they correlate with Patricia Newman's diagnosis of pneumonia.

→ • Click on **Return to Room 406**.
 • Click on **MAR** and select tab **406**.

11. What is the desired therapeutic effect of ipratropium bromide? How could the nurse assess whether the desired effect was achieved?

12. What is the desired therapeutic effect of cefotetan? How could the nurse assess whether the desired effect was achieved?

13. What is the rationale for administration of IV fluids related to pneumonia?

Follow the steps below to prepare and administer the appropriate medication(s) to Patricia Newman.

Medication Preparation

- Click on **Medication Room**.
- Click on **MAR** to determine medications that Patricia Newman is ordered to receive at 0800 and any appropriate prn medications you may want to administer. (*Note:* You may click on **Review MAR** at any time to verify correct medication order. Remember to look at the patient name on the MAR to make sure you have the correct patient's record—you must click on the correct room number within the MAR.) Click on **Return to Medication Room** after reviewing the correct MAR.
- Click on **Unit Dosage**. When the close-up view appears, click on drawer **406**.
- Select the medication(s) you plan to administer. After each medication you select, click **Put Medication on Tray**. When you are finished, click on **Close Drawer**.
- Click **View Medication Room**.
- Click on **IV Storage**. From the close-up view, click on the drawer labeled **Large Volume**.
- Select the medication(s) you plan to administer, put medication(s) on the tray, and then close the bin.
- Click **View Medication Room**.
- Click on **Preparation**. Select the correct medication to administer; click **Prepare** and **Next**.
- Choose the correct patient to administer this medication to and click **Finish**.
- Repeat the above two steps until all medications that you want to administer are prepared.
- You can click **Review Your Medications** and then **Return to Medication Room** when ready. From the Medication Room, you may go directly to Patricia Newman's room by clicking on **406** at the bottom of the screen.

Medication Administration

- Administer the medication, utilizing the five rights of medication administration. After you have collected the appropriate assessment data and are ready for administration, click **Patient Care** and **Medication Administration**. Verify that the correct patient and medication(s) appear in the left-hand window. Then click the down arrow next to Select. From the drop-down menu, select **Administer** and complete the Administration Wizard by providing any information requested. When the Wizard stops asking for information, click **Administer to Patient**. Specify **Yes** when asked whether this administration should be recorded in the MAR. Finally, click **Finish**.

Check Your Work

- Now let's see how you did! Click on **Leave the Floor** at the bottom of your screen. From the Floor Menu, select **Look at Your Preceptor's Evaluation**. Then click on **Medication Scorecard**.

14. Note below whether or not you correctly administered the appropriate medications. If not, why do you think you were incorrect? According to Table C in this scorecard, what are the appropriate resources that should be used and important assessments that should be completed before administering these medications? Did you use these resources and perform these assessments correctly?

Exercise 3

 CD-ROM Activity

 40 minutes

- Sign in to work at Pacific View Regional Hospital for Period of Care 2. (*Note:* If you are already in the virtual hospital from a previous exercise, click on **Leave the Floor** and then **Restart the Program** to get to the sign-in window.)
- From the Patient List, select Patricia Newman (Room 406).
- Click on **Go to Nurses' Station**.
- Click on **Chart** and then on **406**.
- Click on **History and Physical**.

1. How long ago was Patricia Newman diagnosed with emphysema?

2. What clinical manifestations documented on the H&P can be attributed to emphysema?

3. What additional clinical manifestations might you expect to see in other clients with emphysema?

→ • Click on **Diagnostic Reports**.

4. What findings on the CXR are consistent with the diagnosis of emphysema?

5. What is the relationship between the client's admitting diagnosis (pneumonia) and her underlying chronic condition (emphysema)?

6. What other pulmonary complication of emphysema should the nurse be alert for in Patricia Newman? Explain the pathophysiologic basis for this occurrence.

7. If Patricia Newman would have a 12-lead ECG done, what abnormalities might you expect related to her emphysema?

→ • Click on **Physician's Orders**.

8. What is the order for oxygen?

9. What is the rationale for this oxygen order as opposed to the usual goal of greater than 90%-93% oxygen saturation?

➤ • Click on **Patient Education**.

10. What is educational goal 3 for Patricia Newman?

11. Explain the rationale for using this breathing technique.

12. What is educational goal 4 for Patricia Newman?

13. What do you think Patricia Newman's special dietary needs are? Explain your answer.

14. What is education goal 6 for Patricia Newman?

15. Explain the rationale for using this technique.

16. Since Patricia Newman's emphysema puts her at high risk for pulmonary infections, what would you teach her to do to help prevent further episodes of pneumonia? (*Hint:* See NCP on page 1582 of your textbook.)

- Click on **Return to Nurses' Station** and then on **406** to go to Patricia Newman's room.
- Inside the room, click on **Patient Care** and then on **Nurse-Client Interactions**.
- Select and view the video titled **1100: Care Coordination**. (*Note:* Check the virtual clock to see whether enough time has elapsed. You can use the fast-forward feature to advance the time by 2-minute intervals if the video is not yet available. Then click again on **Patient Care** and **Nurse-Client Interactions** to refresh the screen.)

17. What disciplines are involved in planning and providing care for Patricia Newman? List these below; then explain the role of each discipline in helping meet the client's health care needs.

Involved Disciplines   **Role in Patricia's Health Care**

LESSON **21**

Glaucoma

 Reading Assignment: Management of Clients with Visual Disorders (Chapter 65)

Patient: Clarence Hughes, Room 404

Goal: Use the nursing process to competently care for clients with glaucoma.

Objectives:

1. Describe the pathophysiology of glaucoma.
2. Identify clinical manifestations related to glaucoma.
3. Describe appropriate pharmacologic treatment of glaucoma.
4. Administer eyedrops safely and accurately.
5. Evaluate a client's ability to correctly administer prescribed ophthalmic medication.

Overview:

In this lesson you will learn the essentials of caring for a client diagnosed with glaucoma. You will explore the client's history, evaluate presenting symptoms and treatment, administer prescribed medications, and develop an individualized discharge teaching plan. Clarence Hughes is a 73-year-old male admitted for an elective left knee arthroplasty.

Exercise 1

 Clinical Preparation: Writing Activity

15 minutes

1. Describe the pathophysiology of glaucoma.

2. Identify and describe the two major types of glaucoma.

3. Identify factors associated with the development of open-angle glaucoma.

Exercise 2

  CD-ROM Activity

45 minutes

- Sign in to work at Pacific View Regional Hospital for Period of Care 3. (*Note:* If you are already in the virtual hospital from a previous exercise, click on **Leave the Floor** and then **Restart the Program** to get to the sign-in window.)
- From the Patient List, select Clarence Hughes (Room 404).
- Click on **Go to Nurses' Station**.
- Click on **Chart** and then on **404**.
- Click on **History and Physical**.

1. What problems of the eye does Clarence Hughes have?

2. How would this be diagnosed? Briefly explain the procedure and expected results. (Hint: See page 1687 of your textbook.)

3. What signs and symptoms do you think Clarence Hughes had prior to diagnosis?

4. For what clinical manifestation(s) and/or history should you assess Clarence Hughes related to this diagnosis?

5. The History and Physical does not identify the type of glaucoma Clarence Hughes has. Based on his history and the information in your textbook, which type do you think Clarence Hughes most likely has? Explain why you came to this conclusion.

• Click on **Return to Nurses' Station**.
• Click on **MAR** and then on **404**.

6. What medications are ordered for Clarence Hughes' glaucoma? Identify these medications, their classifications, and mechanisms of action below. You will complete the last column in question 7. (*Hint:* You may consult the Drug Guide in the Nurses' Station.)

Medication	Drug Classification	Mechanism of Action	Side Effects

7. For what side effects should you monitor Clarence Hughes related to these medications? Record your answer in the table in question 6.

8. If you were to administer the prescribed antiglaucoma medication to Clarence Hughes, how would you correctly apply the eye drops? Explain the step-by-step procedure. (*Hint:* Consult the Drug Guide by clicking on the **Drug** icon in the lower left corner of your screen.)

9. What would you expect Clarence Hughes' tonometry reading to be prior to beginning treatment for glaucoma? What would you expect the reading to be during treatment?

10. Identify an appropriate outcome for Clarence Hughes related to his glaucoma.

→ • Click on **Return to Nurses' Station**.
   • Click on **Chart** and then on **404**.
   • Click on **Patient Education**.

11. What educational goals would you add for Clarence Hughes related to his glaucoma?

12. What teaching would you provide for Clarence Hughes regarding his glaucoma?

13. Complete the following table by documenting the teaching points you would review with Clarence Hughes regarding his glaucoma medications. (*Hint:* Consult the Drug Guide.)

Medication	Teaching Points

14. What teaching methods would you use to teach medication administration?

15. How would you evaluate Clarence Hughes' understanding of correct application?

16. If Clarence Hughes' ophthalmic medications fail to maintain his IOP within normal limits, what other therapy might he expect to undergo? Briefly explain these procedures.

LESSON **22** ——————————————————————

Low Back Pain

————————————————————————————————

✐ **Reading Assignment:** Management of Clients with Peripheral Nervous System
Disorders (Chapter 71)

Patient: Jacquline Catanazaro, Room 402

Goal: Use the nursing process to competently care for clients with an intervertebral disk
problem.

Objectives:

1. Describe the pathophysiology of low back pain.
2. Identify clinical manifestations related to low back pain and/or herniated intervertebral disk.
3. Plan appropriate interventions to treat low back pain.
4. Evaluate a client's potential to comply with a health care management plan.
5. Develop an individualized teaching plan for a client with low back pain.

Overview:

In this lesson you will learn the essentials of caring for a client experiencing chronic low back
pain. You will explore the client's history, evaluate presenting symptoms and treatment, plan
appropriate nursing interventions to treat the client's symptoms, and develop an individualized
discharge teaching plan. Jacquline Catanazaro is a 45-year-old female admitted with an acute
exacerbation of asthma.

Exercise 1

 Clinical Preparation: Writing Activity

 10 minutes

1. Describe the underlying pathophysiology of low back pain.

2. Define the following procedures.

   a. Microdiskectomy

   b. Decompressive laminectomy

   c. Artificial disk replacement

   d. Spinal fusion (arthodesis)

Exercise 2

 CD-ROM Activity

 45 minutes

- Sign in to work at Pacific View Regional Hospital for Period of Care 3. (*Note:* If you are already in the virtual hospital from a previous exercise, click on **Leave the Floor** and then **Restart the Program** to get to the sign-in window.)
- From the Patient List, select Jacquline Catanazaro (Room 402).
- Click on **Go to Nurses' Station**.
- Click on **Chart** and then on **402**.
- Click on **History and Physical**.

1. Under "History of Present Illness," what are Jacquline Catanazaro's complaints related to her back?

2. How does the physician describe this problem under "Past Medical History"?

3. How was this diagnosed?

4. How long has she had this problem?

5. What treatment has she undergone? Explain the mechanism of action and/or rationale for these treatments.

6. What "red flag" conditions(s) does Jacquline Catanazaro have that could be associated with her low back pain?

7. What assessment should be completed on Jacquline Catanazaro in relation to the back pain?

→ • Click on **Nurse's Notes**.

8. How have the nurses addressed Jacquline Catanazaro's complaints of low back pain?

9. What interventions can you suggest that would be appropriate to control Jacquline Catanazaro's pain?

 • Click on **History and Physical**.

 10. What is the physician's plan regarding the client's back pain? What type of interventions might be offered by this plan? (*Hint:* See Chapter 20 of your textbook.)

11. What interventions would you plan to improve Jacquline Catanazaro's mobility and thus her activity level?

12. If Jacquline Catanazaro's back pain persists with the current medical management, does research support the use of surgical therapy to improve her clinical outcome?

13. If Jacquline Catanazaro would decide to undergo surgery in an effort to find pain relief, for what potential postoperative problems/complications would you need to monitor her?

→ • Click on **Patient Education**.

14. What goals related to Jacquline Catanazaro's back pain would you add?

15. Develop a discharge teaching plan for Jacquline Catanazaro to help relieve and prevent further back pain. (*Hint:* See Client Education Guide for Lower Back Care on the Evolve site.)

→ • Click on **History and Physical**.

16. What may interfere with Jacquline Catanazaro's compliance to health care instructions?

- Click on **Return to Nurses' Station**.
- Click on **402** to enter Jacquline Catanazaro's room.
- Click on **Patient Care** and then on **Nurse-Client Interactions**.
- Select and view the video titled **1540: Discharge Planning**. (*Note:* Check the virtual clock to see whether enough time has elapsed. You can use the fast-forward feature to advance the time by 2-minute intervals if the video is not yet available. Then click again on **Patient Care** and **Nurse-Client Interactions** to refresh the screen.)

17. After viewing the video, what other suggestions do you have for assisting Jacquline Catanazaro with compliance after discharge? (*Hint:* See Chapter 1 in your textbook.)

LESSON **23** _____

Blood Component Therapy

_____

⟲ Reading Assignment: Management of Clients with Hematologic Disorders
(Chapter 75)

Patient: Piya Jordan, Room 403

Goal: Use the nursing process to competently care for clients receiving various blood
products.

Objectives:

1. Describe the ABO and Rh antigen systems.
2. Identify the correct type blood to administer to a specific client.
3. Describe appropriate nursing responsibilities related to blood product administration.
4. Evaluate vital sign assessments related to potential blood transfusion reactions.
5. Describe appropriate assessment parameters when monitoring for various types of transfusion reactions.

Overview:

In this lesson you will learn the essentials of caring for a client receiving blood and blood product transfusions. You will describe pretransfusion responsibilities, identify administration
specifics, and evaluate the client during and after each transfusion. Piya Jordan is a 68-year-old
female admitted with nausea, vomiting, and abdominal pain.

Exercise 1

 Clinical Preparation: Writing Activity

 10 minutes

 1. Describe the ABO antigen system. (*Hint:* Read page 1991 of your textbook.)

2. Describe the Rh antigen system.

 3. Complete the following table to identify which types of blood are compatible with each other. (*Hint:* Use Table 75-1 in your textbook.)

Client's Blood Type	Blood Types That This Client May Receive
A+	
A–	
B+	
B–	
O+	
O–	
AB+	
AB–	

Exercise 2

 CD-ROM Activity

 30 minutes

- Sign in to work at Pacific View Regional Hospital for Period of Care 1. (*Note:* If you are already in the virtual hospital from a previous exercise, click on **Leave the Floor** and then **Restart the Program** to get to the sign-in window.)
- From the Patient List, select Piya Jordan (Room 403).
- Click on **Go to Nurses' Station**.
- Click on **Chart** and then on **403**.
- Click on **Laboratory Reports**.

1. Record Piya Jordan's hematology results below.

	Monday 2200	Tuesday 0630	Wednesday 0630
Hemoglobin			
Hematocrit			

2. Why do you think Piya Jordan's H&H is lower on Wednesday? (*Hint:* Check the Physican's Notes in the chart.)

→ - Click on **Physician's Orders**.

3. What was ordered to address the client's H&H results? Is this appropriate related to Piya Jordan's level of hemoglobin? Explain why or why not.

• Click on **Return to Nurses' Station** and then on **403** to enter Piya Jordan's room.

• Click on **Patient Care** and then on **Nurse-Client Interactions**.

• Select and view the video titled **0735: Pain—Adverse Drug Event**. (*Note:* Check the virtual clock to see whether enough time has elapsed. You can use the fast-forward feature to advance the time by 2-minute intervals if the video is not yet available. Then click again on **Patient Care** and **Nurse-Client Interactions** to refresh the screen.)

4. What does the nurse state she will do to prepare Piya Jordan for a blood transfusion?

5. What gauge IV would you insert to best ensure maximal flow rate of undiluted RBCs?

 • Click on **Chart** and then on **403**.

• Click on **Laboratory Reports**.

6. What pretransfusion testing must be completed to ensure compatability of blood with the client? Are these documented on Piya Jordan's chart?

7. What other pretransfusion responsibilities would you complete prior to requesting blood release?

8. What must the client sign prior to receiving the ordered blood? Did Piya Jordan sign it? If so, where can you locate it on her chart?

9. What type of administration sets could you use for blood products.

Exercise 3

 CD-ROM Activity

 30 minutes

- Sign in to work at Pacific View Regional Hospital for Period of Care 2. (*Note:* If you are already in the virtual hospital from a previous exercise, click on **Leave the Floor** and then **Restart the Program** to get to the sign-in window.)
- From the Patient List, select Piya Jordan (Room 403).
- Click on **Go to Nurses' Station**.
- Click on **403** to enter Piya Jordan's room.
- Click on **Patient Care** and then **Nurse-Client Interactions**.
- Select and view the video titled **1115: Interventions—Nausea and Blood**. (*Note:* Check the virtual clock to see whether enough time has elapsed. You can use the fast-forward feature to advance the time by 2-minute intervals if the video is not yet available. Then click again on **Patient Care** and **Nurse-Client Interactions** to refresh the screen.)

1. Piya Jordan's daughter voices concern regarding the safety of blood transfusion. How did the nurse respond to this?

2. Describe how you would explain the safety of blood transfusions.

3. During the video, the nurse states that the blood has just arrived. How soon should the nurse begin the transfusion?

→ • Click on **Chart** and then on **403**.
   • Click on **Laboratory Reports**.

4. What is Piya Jordan's blood type?

5. What type of blood may she receive safely?

6. Describe the nurse's responsibilities during the initiation of this transfusion.

7. What assessments should be completed on Piya Jordan during the transfusion?

8. What would you do if Piya Jordan displayed any unusual manifestations during the blood transfusion?

9. What would you document regarding this blood transfusion?